COVID-19
aTCM
Perspective

COVID-19
aTCM
Perspective

温故知新——中医论新冠

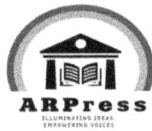

ARPress
ILLUMINATING IDEAS.
EMPOWERING VOICES

Shiwu Xiao M.D. (China), L.Ac., M.S.O.M

Baisong Zhong M.D. (China), Ph.D, L.Ac.

Michael Johnston L.Ac., M.S.O.M.

Daohe Fang M.D. (China), L.Ac., M.S.O.M.

Ding Ding M.D. (China)

ARPress
45 Dan Road Suite 5
Canton MA 02021

Hotline: 1(888) 821-0229
Fax: 　　1(508) 545-7580

Ordering Information:
Quantity sales. Special discounts are available on quantity purchases by corporations, associations, and others. For details, contact the publisher at the address above.

Printed in the United States of America.

ISBN-13: 　　　Paperback　　　979-8-89356-381-8
　　　　　　　　eBook　　　　　979-8-89356-380-1

Library of Congress Control Number: 2024903073

Table of Contents

Preface

The world has been shocked and people's general lives has been severely affected by Covid-19 since 2019 because there has been no clear Western drugs or pharmaceuticals that can cure Covid-19. There has been no effective therapies to reduce complications and fatalities of Covid-19, even though scientists from all walks of life are trying to explore effective ways to cure it. As Traditional Chinese medical practitioners, we treat a large number of patients whose diseases relate to Covid-19, including before, during and, after Covid-19. With the efforts of many Traditional Chinese Medicine (TCM) medical staff, we have used traditional Chinese herbs, acupuncture, and other TCM therapies to prevent and treat Covid-19. I'm glad to say that we achieved impressive results. Together, Chinese, and Western medicine experts have practiced, done research and taught people about TCM for more than thirty years and have contributed to this book about treating Covid-19 with TCM. This book is the most practical reference ever written for licensed acupuncturists, TCM students, researchers, and other medical practitioners to understand, prevent and treat Covid-19 with Traditional Chinese Medicine.

Chapter One, "Introduction to Covid-19 and History of Pandemic Diseases". The first part contains new information about mechanism of onset, spread of Covid-19, and research on Covid-19. The second part describes the TCM History on plagues. It serves as a comprehensive introduction or basic understanding of plagues by TCM. Prevention methods for pandemic diseases, such as the earliest anti-serum therapy and vaccines, and classic treatments for pandemic diseases, such as therapies of Shang Han Za Bing Lun (Treatise on Cold Pathogenic and Miscellaneous Diseases) and Wen Bing (Warmth Induced Disorders).

Chapter Two, "TCM Prevention and Management of COVID-19". A new chapter on the preventive treatment focuses not only on the importance of expelling toxins of Covid-19, but also on the risk factors that create susceptible physical constitutions. It also gives us handy, easy and practical precautions.

Chapter Three, "TCM Treatment During COVID-19". This chapter provides new therapies from the theory of six meridians syndrome differentiation, the Wei, Qi, Ying, and Blood theory, and San Jiao differentiation as well as treating Covid-19. We also added new ideas for treating severe complications of Covid-19 with our clinic experience.

Chapter Four, " TCM Treatment of Post COVID-19". This chapter focuses on classic TCM therapies for common symptoms after suffering from Covid-19, such as brain fog, anxiety, lost taste and smell, shortness of breath, body pain, PTSD and fatigue post Covid-19, also for disorders of the five Zang-Fu organs post Covid-19, which are the Heart, Liver, Spleen, Stomach, Lung and Kidney.

Chapter Five, "Research of Covid-19 in TCM". This chapter is completely filled with research of new therapies to treat Covid-19 with TCM. It makes acupuncture and herbs more advanced. It also adds a new Diagnosis and Treatment Protocol for Covid-19.

The first and third chapters in this book are written by Dr. Shiwu Xiao L.Ac, MD (China), Dr. Ding Ding MD (China) and Michael Johnston L.Ac. The second, fourth and five chapters by Dr. Baisong Zhong, L.Ac, Ph.D, MD (China) and Dr. Daohe Fang L.Ac, MD (China). Michael Johnston's many contributions to this book were enhanced by his clear writing and editing skills that permitted him to distill complex concepts into easily readable prose accessible to a general medical readership.

We wish to express our appreciation to our many associates and colleagues, who, as experts in their fields, have helped us with constructive criticism and helpful suggestions.

Baisong Zhong L.Ac, Ph.D, MD (China)

Chapter One

Introduction

Covid 19, officially termed as SARS CoV-2 is the largest pandemic affecting people across all borders and demographics in modern history. At the time of the writing of this book there are 116,942,106 active cases of Covid 19 and 2,595,106 deaths. There are currently 60,000 new cases every day, however death rates have decreased significantly. Researchers credit several factors contributing to this positive shift. There has been no clear treatment, drug, or therapy that we can assign as a standalone reason for reduced fatalities, rather a combination of factors. These include a better understanding of the virus and how it responds to available treatments, an overall decrease in the number of cases which has taken intense pressure off healthcare systems, and physicians are getting better at treating Covid-19 patients. These are just a couple of the possible contributing factors. The overall effectiveness of vaccines is yet to be fully understood as new variants of the virus emerge along with the loosening of restrictions in many regions.

Earliest cases were reported in Wuhan, China. One common denominator amongst the early cases was that several people had visited a Wuhan meat and animal market, it is not understood what role this market played in any insemination or spread of covid 19. Samples taken from drains and sewage did test positive for the virus however, no significant leads have caused researchers and investigators to be able to narrow down to a credible and actual source.

The WHO team is currently trying to cover all angles in terms of discovering how and where Covid 19 started. This includes visiting multiple animal markets around China, surveying multiple animal species that would be most likely to carry SARS-CoV-2 as well as tracing the routes these various species may have traveled. The team is performing contact tracing with the people first-known to have contracted Covid 19, they are testing the medical staff who treated them. They are taking blood samples from laboratory technicians, farm workers and anyone thought to have developed anti-bodies.

A WHO article dated March 2020 states "It is not possible to determine precisely how humans in China were initially infected with SARS-CoV-2. However, all available evidence suggests that SARS-CoV-2 has a natural animal origin and is not a manipulated or constructed virus. SARS-CoV-2 virus most probably has its ecological reservoir in bats."

The origin of an epidemic is extremely laborious and oftentimes unfruitful no matter how rigorous an attempt is mounted; a pandemic is exponentially harder. There are multiple obstacles preventing the collection of relevant and clean data. These include how well information was collected at all stages of time throughout the event, regional and geopolitical relationships, and willingness of various governments to divulge and share important information. Since December 2019, it is well known that the sensitivity of international relationships and the actions of multiple national leaders strained the free exchange of information and likely impinged on the investigation at a critical time.

The Biomedical Journal in August of 2020 reported the "All human coronaviruses have animal origins, namely, natural hosts. Bats may be the natural hosts of HCoV-229E, SARS-CoV, HCoV-NL63, and MERS-CoV. Furthermore, HCoV-OC43 and HKU1 probably originated from rodents. Bats are undoubtedly important and the major natural reservoirs of alpha-coronaviruses and beta-coronaviruses. Domestic animals can suffer from disease as intermediate hosts that cause virus transmission from natural hosts to humans; for example, SARS-CoV and MERS-CoV crossed the species barriers into masked palm civets and camels, respectively. SARS-CoV-2 sequenced at the early stage of the COVID-19 outbreak only shares 79.6% sequence identity with SARS-CoV through early full-length genomic comparisons. However, it is highly identical (96.2%) at the whole-genome level to Bat-CoV RaTG13, which was previously detected in *Rhinolophus affinis* from Yunnan Province, over 1500 km from Wuhan. Bats are likely reservoir hosts for SARS-CoV-2; however, whether Bat-CoV RaTG13 directly jumped to humans or transmits to intermediate hosts to facilitate animal-to-human transmission remains inconclusive. No intermediate host sample was obtained by scientists in an initial cluster of infections of the Huanan Seafood and Wildlife Market in Wuhan, where the sale of wild animals may be the source of zoonotic infection. Furthermore, the earliest three patients with symptom onset had no known history of exposure to the Huanan market. Therefore, there may be multiple sources of COVID-19 in the beginning. According to previous studies by metagenomic sequencing for the samples from Malayan pangolins (Manis javanica) in Guangxi and Guangdong, China, it has been suggested that pangolins might be the intermediate hosts between bats and humans because of the similarity of the pangolin coronavirus to SARS-CoV-2. However, the additional phylogenetic analyses effectively trace COVID-19 infection sources. In addition to the zoonotic origins of SARS-CoV-2 by natural evolution, there are still some disputes about the origin of the virus because its spike protein seems to perfectly interact with the human receptor in contributing to human-to-human transmission after evolution in a short period. Nevertheless, more direct evidence is required to clarify the arguments."

Nevertheless, no author of this book is an epidemiologist or member of the WHO team investigating the inception of Covid 19. While we are interested in understanding the how and why and where Covid 19 started in the spirit of prevention and management of future pandemics, this book will focus on presenting information about the virus, how it is spread and how to treat its various stages from a Traditional Chinese Medicine perspective.

Onset

Coronavirus disease 2019 (Covid-19) is defined as illness caused by a novel coronavirus now called severe acute respiratory syndrome coronavirus 2 (SARS-CoV-2; formerly called 2019-nCoV) which was first identified amid an outbreak of respiratory illness cases in Wuhan City, Hubei Province, China. SARS-CoV-2 is believed to be a spillover of an animal coronavirus and later adapted the ability of human-to-human transmission.

Coronavirus disease SARS-CoV-2 has had a global impact. It is the fifth pandemic after the 1918 flu pandemic. As of now, we can trace the first report and subsequent outbreak from a cluster of novel human pneumonia cases in Wuhan City, China, since late December 2019. The earliest date of symptom onset was 1 December 2019. Initially, the disease was called Wuhan pneumonia by the press because of the area and pneumonia symptoms. Covid-19 is the seventh member of the coronavirus family to infect humans. On 11 March 2020, the WHO finally made the assessment that COVID-19 can be characterized as a pandemic.

SARS-CoV-2 began like all new viruses with an ordinary moment when a cluster of patients admitted to a hospital with pneumonia turned out to have a new strain of coronavirus. The virus's high transmissibility made the epidemic in China turn into a global pandemic with an ongoing daily reporting of new cases and deaths. However, as fast as viruses spread, the detection of pandemics and taking early measures has become much easier due to the advancement of science in today's world. The early responses and measures adopted by China, such as early reporting and situation monitoring, large-scale surveillance, and preparation of medical facilities and supplies, were all successful in reducing the epidemic in China generally and in the epicenter Wuhan specifically.

A 2020 Dubai medical journal wrote "To look for the infection source, authorities started their surveillance with investigating food markets other than the Huanan Seafood market. As for infected patients, clinical case identification was provided by WHO China and CDC China to have clear criteria for identifying cases under the outbreak investigation. The national authorities later placed public health strategies and follow-ups for cases and contacts, and more than 1,800 teams of epidemiologists were assigned to trace tens of thousands of people a day in Wuhan. In addition, a community-wide temperature screening was implemented through "installing infrared thermometers in airports, railway stations, long-distance bus stations, and ferry terminals". Thousands of health and quarantine stations were also set up in national service areas and in entrances and exits for passengers at stations. The search was later expanded to include screening people at work, in shops and on streets. Furthermore, the government followed more aggressive ways of health checking by sending officials to residents' houses and forcing ill people to be isolated.

The Chinese government has been investing in new high technology tracking systems as well. One example is the smartphone application which is based on a health code color system that categorizes individuals into three color groups based on their health status and travel history, and then determine whether they need to be quarantined. Another measure that helped in disease surveillance and controlling is the street camera system that can catch, and fine individuals walking publicly without a mask and identify those showing symptoms. This system is known to be effective as it was previously used during the SARS outbreak but recently updated to include facial recognition and to cover all areas in China."

The Centers for Disease Control and Prevention has estimated that SARS-CoV-2 entered the United States in late January or early February, establishing low-level community spread before being noticed. On April 3, 2020, the CDC issued a recommendation that the general public, even those without symptoms, should begin wearing face coverings in public settings where social-distancing measures are difficult to maintain in order to abate the spread of COVID-19.

Spread

The coronavirus is thought to have spread mainly from person to person. This can happen between people who are in close contact with one another. Close contact is typically considered to be 6 feet apart or less. Droplets that are produced when an infected person coughs or sneezes may land in the mouths or noses of people who are nearby, or possibly be inhaled into their Lungs. A person infected with coronavirus — even one with no symptoms — may emit aerosols when they talk, breathe, cough or sneeze. Aerosols are infectious viral particles that can float or drift around in the air for up to three hours. Another person may breathe in these aerosols and become infected with the coronavirus. Therefore, everyone should cover their nose and mouth when they go out in public.

Coronavirus can also spread from contact with infected surfaces or objects. For example, a person can get COVID-19 by touching a surface or object that has the virus on it and then touching their own mouth, nose, or possibly their eyes. Coronavirus may live on surfaces from hours to days. Sunlight and heat will reduce the length of time the virus can survive on surfaces. The virus may be shed in saliva, semen, and feces. Kissing can transmit the virus. Transmission of the virus through feces or sexual contact appears to be extremely unlikely. Like other viruses, SARS-CoV-2 cannot survive without a living cell in which to reproduce. Once it enters human cells, SARS-CoV-2 makes copies of itself, which go on to infect other cells. Sometimes, a mistake is made when the virus is replicating. This is called a mutation. Mutations have led to two new coronavirus variants. One, called B.1.1.7, was first detected in the United Kingdom. The other, called B.1.351, originated in South Africa. Both variants have now been detected in countries around the globe. Both variants contain mutations on the virus's spike protein. Spike proteins on the surface of the SARS-CoV-2 virus bind to and allow the virus to enter human cells. Interestingly, both variants share a key mutation (called N501Y) on the spike protein, that allows the virus to bind more tightly to human cells. This mutation makes the new variants more contagious than previous SARS-CoV-2 variants. But they do not appear to be deadlier than other variants. The emergence of these highly transmissible variants is yet another reason why mask wearing, physical distancing, and avoiding crowds continues to be as important as ever.

The table below shows data collected at Johns Hopkins University

World

Infections 91,602,686

Fatalities 1,961,455

United States
22,838,110
380,670
India
10,495,147
151,529
Brazil
8,195,637
204,690
Russia
3,412,390
61,908
United Kingdom
3,164,051
83,203
France
2,800,770
68,431
Turkey
2,346,285
23,152
Italy
2,303,263
79,819
Spain
2,137,220
52,683

Germany
1,968,326
42,889
Colombia
1,816,082
46,782
Argentina
1,744,704
44,848
Mexico
1,556,028
135,682
Poland
1,395,779
31,593
Iran
1,299,022
56,360
South Africa
1,259,748
34,334
Ukraine
1,160,243
20,915
Peru
1,037,350
38,335
Netherlands
883,135
12,563
Indonesia
846,765
24,645

Source: Center for Systems Science and Engineering at Johns Hopkins University

Anyone who comes into close contact with someone who has COVID-19 is at increased risk of becoming infected themselves, and of potentially infecting others. Contact tracing can help prevent further transmission of the virus by quickly identifying and informing people who may be infected and contagious, so they can take steps to not infect others. Contact tracing begins with identifying everyone that a person recently diagnosed with COVID-19 has been in contact with since they became contagious. In the case of COVID-19, a person may be contagious 48 to 72 hours before they start to experience symptoms. The contacts are notified about their exposure. CDC protocols advise people who have come into close contact with a person infected with Covid-19 to quarantine themselves for 14 days, watch for fever or shortness of breath and try to limit contact with other people in the home. Close contact includes being within 6 ft of an infected person for longer than 15 minutes, providing home care to a person with Covid-19, direct physical contact with the person such as kissing or hugging, sharing eating or drinking utensils, or somehow coming into contact with their respiratory droplets.

Future

At the time of this writing 4 vaccines have been deployed internationally. Vaccines are weakened or dead parts of pathogenic material. Vaccines train our immune system to recognize these pathogens so that if a pathogen enters our system, we can produce appropriate antibodies to fight it. Vaccinations vary greatly in their effectiveness. At best, they can offer the opportunity of not catching an infectious disease. Down from that, they may prevent a vaccinated person from getting a full-blown infection and/ or reducing their potency of transmission. The vaccine for Covid-19 is indeed unique. Typically, vaccine development takes years, even decades before they are ready for use. It took the FDA less than one year to grant Emergency Use Authorization for two vaccines, Pfizer and Moderna. Two others, Astra-Zeneca and Johnson and Johnson are also being utilized and several others are on the way.

A November 2020 BBC website reported "The biggest misconception is the work on the vaccine started when the pandemic began. The world's biggest Ebola outbreak in 2014-2016 was a catastrophe. The response was too slow, and 11,000 people died. In the recriminations that followed, a plan emerged for how to tackle the next big one. At the end of a list of known threats was "Disease X" - the sinister name of a new, unknown infection that would take the world by surprise. The Jenner Institute at the University of Oxford - named after the scientist that performed the first vaccination in 1796, and now home to some of the world's leading experts - designed a strategy for defeating an unknown enemy.

The central piece of their plan was a revolutionary style of vaccine known as "plug and play". It has two highly desirable traits for facing the unknown - it is both fast and flexible.

Conventional vaccines - including the whole of the childhood immunization program - use a killed or weakened form of the original infection or inject fragments of it into the body. But these are slow to develop. Instead, the Oxford researchers constructed ChAdOx1 - or Chimpanzee Adenovirus Oxford One. Scientists took a common cold virus that infected chimpanzees and engineered it to become the building block of a vaccine against almost anything. Before Covid, 330 people had been given ChAdOx1 based vaccines for diseases ranging from flu to Zika virus, and prostate cancer to the tropical disease chikungunya. The virus from chimps is genetically modified so it cannot cause an infection in people. It can then be modified again to contain the genetic blueprints for whatever you want to train the immune system to attack. This target is known as an antigen. ChAdOx1 is in essence a sophisticated, microscopic postman. All the scientists have to do is change the package. "We drop it in and off we go," said Prof Gilbert. While much of the world was having a lie-in after New Year's Eve, Prof Gilbert noticed concerning reports of "viral pneumonia" in Wuhan, China. Within two weeks scientists had identified the virus responsible and began to suspect it was able to spread between people.

"We'd been planning for disease X, we'd been waiting for disease X, and I thought this could be it," Prof Gilbert said. At this point, the team did not know how important their work would become. It started out as a test of how fast they could go and as a demonstration of the ChAdOx1 technology.

Prof Gilbert said: "I thought it might only have been a project, we'd make the vaccine and the virus would fizzle out. But it did not. It sounds strange to say it, almost perverse, but it was lucky that the pandemic was caused by a coronavirus.

This family of viruses had tried to jump from animals to people twice before in the past 20 years - SARS coronavirus in 2002 and MERS coronavirus in 2012. It meant scientists knew the virus's biology, how it behaved and its Achilles heel - the "spike protein".

As previously mentioned, vaccines typically use weakened or dead parts of pathogens to teach the body to recognize and fight infectious invasions. However, another unique aspect of the Covid-19 pandemic is the utilization of an mRNA vaccine. These kinds of vaccine are new but are not unknown. mRNA vaccine research has been going for decades and from a research and manufacturing standpoint they are superior to more traditional vaccines. They can be formulated using readily available resources and can be scaled up for manufacture much quicker. The mRNA gives our cells instructions to make a spike protein, like the spike protein found on the surface of Covid-19. Once that protein is manufactured by our own cells, our immune system begins to recognize it as "other" and mounts an immune response against it.

Again, from Oxford university "We had a huge head start," Prof Andrew Pollard from the Oxford team said. The spike protein is the key the virus uses to unlock the doorway into our body's cells. If a vaccine could train the immune system to attack the spike, then the team knew they were odds-on to succeed.

And they had already developed a ChAdOx1 vaccine for MERS which could train the immune system to spot the spike. The Oxford team were not starting from scratch. It was also lucky that coronaviruses cause short-term infections. It means the body can beat the virus and a vaccine just needs to tap into that natural process. If it had been a long-term or chronic infection that the body cannot beat - like HIV - then it's unlikely a vaccine could work. On 11 January, Chinese scientists published and shared with the world the full genetic code of the coronavirus. The team now had everything they needed to make a Covid-19 vaccine. All they had to do was slip the genetic instructions for the spike protein into ChAdOx1 and they were good to go."

All vaccines then had to complete the standard 3-phase trials to prove safety and efficacy. All aspects have been expedited from funding to production to regulation and distribution. According to industry standards all elements of safety and proper protocol have been summarily satisfied. Much of the "red tape" has been cut in order make these vaccines available as the pandemic continued to spread.

In the U.S. the rollout has been clunky. There has been several instances of feast and famine, lacking equitable and widespread distribution. Despite poor organization and bad actors on many sides vaccination presses on. On March 10, 2021, Bloomberg news reported "The biggest vaccination campaign in history is underway. More than 321 million doses have been administered across 118 countries. The latest rate was roughly 8.31 million doses a day. In the U.S. more Americans have received at least one dose than have tested positive for the virus since the pandemic began. So far, 95.7 million doses have been given. In the last week, an average of 2.17 million doses per day were administered.

Problems have arisen and will continue to arise. There have been adverse events, there have been numerous conflicting reports about efficacy and side effects. Statistically the numbers report the vaccines to be safe at this point. Reports of adverse events continue to come in, reports of vaccinated people contracting Covid-19 continue to come in. Whether or not these statistics compare reasonably with other vaccines will not be our focus here, time will tell that story.

Considering all of this, the need for a broad-based approach to treatment and prevention has never been more critical. Covid-19 is not over by a long shot and there will be future pandemics. Putting all our eggs in one basket is a myopic and dangerous approach. We need all of the tools available. TCM is well-versed in the treatment of infectious disease. Chinese scientists have meticulously documented pandemics for thousands of years. They have applied intricate systems of diagnosis and treatment of several pandemics and that information is available, and it is relevant in our modern setting. Infectious disease is a theater in which the co-application of Western medicine and TCM can operate very effectively together.

Retrospective History of TCM Epidemiology

According to studies in Wuhan city, Hubei province, China, where COVID- 19 was first discovered, Traditional Chinese Medicine as a conventional medicine in China, has been used successfully in more than 90.6% of all patients there who suffered from COVID- 19. Good therapeutic effects totaling more than 90% [1] have been found in the following aspects-

- TCM herbal prescriptions have been found to be effective at alleviating fever, shortness of breath and phlegm accumulation.
- Formulas improve general conditions: treat fatigue and headache, body aches etc.
- Shown antiviral, anti- inflammatory, and antitoxin properties.
- TCM formulas have been found to be effective at improving blood capillary circulation, anti-coagulation and anti-shock mechanisms, therefore protecting multiple inner organs, preventing organ function failure, preventing disease progression and decreasing mortality rates.
- TCM formulas have been found to be effective at increasing the likelihood of negative prognosis, reducing disease rebound and preventing the development of chronicity.
- TCM formulas have been found to be effective at treating sequelae such as pulmonary fibrosis, arrhythmias etc.
- TCM treatment has also been found to be effective at reducing the need for ventilators, ECMO, artificial blood exchange and Lung transplants etc. thereby saving medical resources.
- TCM treatment may also reduce the incidence in affected areas by increasing immunity via the use of immune boosting herbs and by sanitizing the area via the use of herbal air disinfectants.

Since practice in Wu Han, the Chinese government listed TCM in the National COVID-19 prevention and treatment protocol from edition 1-8, applying TCM treatment for millions of people nationwide (91.5%, 74187cases) [2]. Great success has been achieved since then (>90%) [3]. Early intervention of TCM is considerable in improving the cure rate, shortening the course, delaying disease progression, and reducing the mortality rate. [4]

Those successful facts also give rise to the questions of why and how Traditional Chinese Medicine works on COVID-19? Right now there is a lack of approved medications, and vaccinations are just beginning, so called breakthrough cases are found after vaccinations. Seeking effective drugs for COVID-19 including from natural herbs is still an obligate and meaningful task.

We have researched the long history of TCM, and found that it is not a coincidence, it is wisdom from thousands of years of practice and fighting disease, which helped people struggle with epidemics in the past three thousand years. TCM has helped treat SARS, H1N1, COVID-19 in China, it may help to deal with COVID-19 in other parts of the world. Hopefully also for upcoming, unknown epidemics in the future, so called X-diseases (supposed to be less than every five years). This is the initial purpose and significance of writing this book.

As we know, epidemics and infectious diseases have been on the earth far earlier than human beings. We are pretty sure that the fighting between people and diseases started in early human history, correspondingly, in medical science, infectious diseases especially epidemic diseases are always mainstream. It is not an exaggeration to say medical science began and grew along with history as we struggled with epidemic diseases.

Ancient TCM called epidemics as Wen Bing (Warmth induced disorder), when epidemic even pandemic happens, they're called Wen Yi (Plague). As early as the Shang dynasty (BC1250), plague was recorded on Oracle bone scripts, the earliest known form of Chinese writing used on oracle bones—animal bones or turtle plastrons used in pyromantic divination: "sick, no enter", meaning not to approach the sick, because of contagiousness. After studying the Oracle bone script and inscription on ancient bronzeware, archaeologists believe the concept of contagiousness of epidemics and separation measures had already been done during the Shang and Zhou dynasty (BC 1046-256), back then, witchcraft was mixed with medical skill, people thought that diseases were caused by supernatural beings, therefore when epidemics happened, patients were told to dance, pray and perform sacrifice ceremonies to expel diseases.

During the Zhou dynasty, there were already epidemic prevention officers in charge of people's health and year-long epidemic plague prevention work like burning wood to make big fires to expel plague in the city. They periodically emptied and cleared the king's family houses for epidemics. Those activities were recorded in a book by the Zhou Ceremony Regulatory Officer.

Following the Spring Autumn Warring States period, the struggles between TCM and witchcraft reached the apex, historical records (Shiji) recorded the legendary TCM doctor Bian Que (BC407-BC310) refused to treat people who believed in witchcraft, and he was finally killed by witch men. Ultimately TCM prevailed, the milestone marking this was the publication of the TCM bible titled *The Yellow Emperor's Inner Classic*.

The Yellow Emperor's inner classic (Early Qin dynasty-Han dynasty) is the first comprehensive and earliest extant TCM theory book, is also the first book to explore epidemic's aetiology, pathogenesis and treatment principles and even formulas on the following aspects:

(1). The book accurately described the epidemic's characteristics: rapid onset, fast spread, highly contagious, similar symptom presentation, quick development, and how widespread epidemic causes high mortality rates.

Plain questions Chapter72: On acupuncture therapy the Yellow emperor questioned "I heard that when the five plagues come, everyone infected and sick, no matter old or young, all show similar symptoms.

Plain questions Chapter71: The six macrocosmic phases and the six atmospheric influences cause large plagues to come and many people die quickly.

(2). Epidemics are caused by climate abnormalities, related to geographic conditions, and can be predicted by stem and branch theory, the Chinese sexagenary cycle.

(3). Intermediate host description had been observed accurately. The *Yellow Emperor Inner Classic* quoted "Plague could not exist and spread without being hosted by scaled or shelled creatures in rivers and seas, by plume and winged insects or beast, bloody jaundice always brings contagious disease from one either in the water or on earth.

The wild creature lives in a more sophisticated and changing environment, where there are many kinds and different animals live in the same area, therefore it is easier for them to host bacteria and viruses. Protected by creatures, bacteria and viruses constantly survive, evolve and mutate, many develop into new strains of viruses which can infect human beings since there are similarities in the constitution between animals and humans, more than animals to plants.

Now we know that as a matter of fact, more than 70% of human epidemics came from animals, for example: HIV, SARS, Ebola, Bird Flu and swine influenza etc. *The Yellow Emperor Inner Classic* is considered to be the earliest to discover this phenomenon.

(3). Defined epidemics as belonging to heat-type diseases (Febrile disease), to infectious disease, and to Shang Han (cold induced disorder).

Plain questions Chapter31 On heat-type diseases: Nowadays Febrile diseases all belong to Shang Han.[5]

In the Nan Jing, The Yellow Emperor's Eighty-one difficulties classic 58 Shang Han included five kinds: Wind-induced disorder, cold-induced disorder, Warm-dampness, Heat disease, and Warm induced disorders. [6]

(4). Two principles for prevention and treatment: Keep vital qi (strong immunity) and avoid contact (Separation). Emphasis on separation.

Plain questions Chapter72 On acupuncture therapy the Yellow emperor questioned: "I want to know how we can avoid epidemics spreading from person to person". Qi Bo said: "In order to prevent epidemics, first of all keep good vital qi, then evil qi will not enter the body, and avoid contact with toxic qi, especially from entering the nose. Stay away from sick people and spreading will not occur.

The Yellow Emperor's Inner Classic quoted in the Upper Classic "Even in large epidemics, no contact equals no sickness, just keep balance with sufficient defensive Qi".

(5) Created a small gold pill for plague prevention which contains cinnabar, arsenic, found in chapter 71.

(6) Special chapter on Malaria, the earliest in TCM history. chapters 35, 36.

The Yellow Emperor's Inner Classic included epidemics' theoretical groundwork, and directly resulted in the creation of the Shang Han Za Bing Lun (Treatise on Cold Pathogenic and Miscellaneous Diseases). A successful application of the Yellow Emperor's inner Classic theory on diagnosis and treatment of infectious diseases, especially epidemics. The first monograph about this field in TCM and Medical science history.

Not long after the Yellow Emperor Classic, during the East Han Dynasty, Zhang Zhongjing (150-219 A.D.) wrote his book the *Shang Han Za Bing Lun* (Treatise on Cold Pathogenic and Miscellaneous Diseases). It is considered a monument to the understanding and treatment of infectious diseases especially epidemics by TCM. The book explored the regulations of onset, transitions and treatment of cold induced diseases which most commonly occur in Northern China during autumn and winter, mostly influenza, and other epidemics diseases such as acute gastroenteritis, dysentery etc, the main contribution are as following:

(1). Discovered that the common process of those epidemics all go through six stages: starts at Tai Yang superficial stage, then to the Shao Yang stage, then becoming severe in the interior during the Yang Ming stage. First are the three yang meridian stages, then three yin meridian stages, Tai Yin, Shao Yin, Jue Yin, those are more interior levels and can be deadly.

(2). First time recorded the complications of influenza like: most common are acute bronchitis, pneumonia, and bronchial asthma. Severe ones like acute nephritis, myocarditis, pericarditis, reactive thoracicitis, toxic intestinal obstruction, and fatal ones like acute Kidney function failure, shock, Heart failure, and respiratory function failure.

(3). Establishment of the earliest diagnostic method norms in TCM: six meridian differentiation on syndromes system, which become a great tool to analyze and understand epidemics. This book created the most predominant characteristics of TCM, advanced and different from other medical science systems, and for this he became the father of TCM differentiation on syndromes.

(4) Created and recorded a lot of effective formulas as standardized treatments. Unlike his predecessors and peers, instead of using a single herbal formula, Zhang Zhongjing started to use combined formulas, which is more effective while having much less side effects. Proven by almost two thousand years of clinical practice on millions of people, his formulas (314 formulas) have been called classic formulas or experienced formulas. He is considered the father of TCM formulas.

It was Zhang Zhongjing who definitely figured out that febrile diseases, especially epidemics, are the most important doctrine in medical science. Others he called miscellaneous, he advocated elites to study the most advanced compound formulas to fight coming epidemics. Finally he created the Shang Han school and became the most prominent figure in TCM history, being called Medical Sage.

For two thousand years, his formulas have not only been collected as secret in folk, but also been kept in a golden cabinet in the Emperor's Forbidden Palace as the state's most important strategic documents. Later on, this information spread to many Asian countries, and was repeatedly re-edited and published at home and abroad as textbooks by the national health administration in countries like Korea, Japan and Vietnam etc. Since Zhang Zhongjing, TCM started to protect people in East Asia from diseases like influenza by applying formulas like Ma Huang Tang, Gui Zhi Tang and Xiao Chai Hu Tang. For the first time in medical science history doctors were using natural anti-virus, antipyretics and analgesic compound formulas.

We always say that Traditional Chinese Medicine grew to maturity along the struggle in dealing with plagues. Later generations highly regarded his work, even saying Zhang Zhongjing created the laws for all diseases. In modern times, Zhang Zhongjing's six meridian syndrome differentiation and treatment system is still the most important method to analyze, understand and treat epidemics. They have been applied for diseases such as: Measles, Scarlet fever, New influenza like H1N1, SARS etc, especially on current treatment of COVID-19. His system offers significant efficacy, and has been officially recommended in the China National Protocol of Prevention and Treatment of COVID-19 (1st-8th editions). TCM epidemiologists in China even believe that Shang Han Theory is even useful for X-disease in future.

Studies have shown a total of more than 352 recorded plagues have occurred in more than two thousand years in China's history, many because wars between kingdoms caused migration and hunger. Many others may have been due to ethnic integration, commercial exchanges in peacetime, resulting in a growing and concentrated population and the urbanization process. In particular, the northern nomads and the southern farming civilization combined creating the north-south integration, as well as domestic and foreign exchanges.

During the Jin Dynasty, Dr. Gehong (283AD-343AD), wrote *A Handbook of Formulas for Emergencies* he is the originator of First Aid in TCM, it recorded cases of smallpox from captives of the Hun. Before then, the Hun people had struck terror into eastern Europe, spreading this horrible plague. He also recorded the method by applying rabid dog's brain tissues on wounds of patients to treat rabies, and using single sweet wormwood for a malaria treatment. In light of this TCM method, Dr. Tu Youyou from China successfully developed Artemisinin injection, the only effective anti-malaria drug now. This accomplishment gave her the 2015 Nobel Prize in Physiology or Medicine.

Sun Simiao (581AD-682AD), the Emperor's family doctor during the Sui and Tang dynasty, pointed out: Plague and Miasma come from Heaven and Earth, they can be prevented and treated by products of nature. He created a lot of effective formulas for epidemics, recorded in his book *Prescriptions Worth a Thousand Gold for Emergency*, the first medical encyclopaedia, and *The Tang Government Materia Medica*, the first pharmacopeia in history, He was titled as China's King of Medicine for his significant contributions to Chinese Medicine and tremendous care to all patients, old or young, Chinese and foreigners.

Afterwards, the Song dynasty was the most prosperous imperial dynasty in China (960AD-1279AD). The imperial publishing house re-edited *Treatise on Cold Pathogenic and Miscellaneous Diseases* which had been lost for hundreds of years, and the Health administration issued *Formulas Pharmacopeia*. This contained many formulas for plague, like three treasured formulas for unconsciousness due to brain damage: Peace Palace bezoar pill, Blue snow pill and Top treasure pill.

Liu, Wansu, one of the four most predominant TCM doctors in Jin and Yuan Dynasty, stated that all evil qi can finally transform and become interior fire. We should clear interior heat and fire with cool and cold herbs at that stage. He enriched the knowledge about cold-induced plague and enlightened the later generations about Warm-induced plague at the Wen Bing school.

During the Ming Dynasty, the greatest pharmacologist in TCM history Li Shizhen (1518-1593AD) recorded methods for sanitizing the air by steaming vinegar, and disinfecting objects by cooking them in water, earlier than pasteurization created in France, Europe (1862AD).

Unlike the Song dynasty, at the end of Ming dynasty and beginning of Qing Dynasty, doctors started to challenge Shang Han School theory which is more for cold-induced plague, more for Northern area of China along the Yellow River and where the weather is cold. After Qing Manchu conquered China a growing concentration of population and urbanization started, in particular, the northern nomads and the southern farming civilizations. More people live in South China in large cities along the Yangtze River, and the weather is hot. China's population was 150million at the end of the Ming Dynasty, Emperor Qian reached 200 million people, and finally reached 400 million by1833AD. There were more frequent commercial exchanges, plus warm climate, therefore more warm-induced plague appeared.

It was Wu, Youke (1582-1652AD) at the end of Ming Dynasty, who figured out that epidemics are caused not by wind, not by cold, or anything else but evil qi. He also concluded that disease causes differed from humans to animals. Those pathogens enter the human body by breathing through the nose and mouth, his academic viewpoints are the closest to Modern Medical Science. Two hundred years later, with Antonie Leeuwenhoek's invention of the microscope, microbes were first observed in 1828AD. German scientist Christian Ehrenberg named them bacteria. In 1899 AD, viruses were discovered and named. His book *Warm plague treatise* is a milestone and considered the beginning of the Wen Bing school. His formulas like Da Yuan Yin have been popular, even effective for COVID-19.

After Dr. Wu, during the Qing Dynasty in southern China, the Wen Bing school grew rapidly. Representative figures are Dr. Ye Tianshi (1667-1747AD), Xue Shengbai (1681-1770AD), Wu Jutong (1758-1836AD), Wang Mengying (1808-1863AD). These four masters of the Warm induced plague school included spring or summer diseases like influenza, Epidemic Meningitis, Encephalitis, Epidemic Hemorrhagic Fever, Measles, Chickenpox, Scarlet fever Etc, and created the Wei, Qi, Ying, Xue syndrome differentiation and treatment system for Wen Bing and Three Jiao differentiation and treatment system for Damp-heat, the core theories systems of Wen Bing School.

Titled as No. 1 Master of Wen Bing, Ye Tianshi's books *Febrile disease treatise, Clinic Guidance From Cases* are Wen Bing's fundamental theories.

He demonstrated Wen Bing's common aetiology, pathogenesis, routes of contact, location, transmission and prognosis, and principles of treatment, he pointed out that Warm evil qi first attacks the Lungs in the upper part of the body through the mouth and nose. Initially it strikes at the Wei Level, then the Qi level. Many people recover with a desirable prognosis, for seniors or ones with poor constitution, the disease may progress to the Ying and even the Blood level. Bleeding may present, then obstruction syndrome and collapse syndrome and an adverse prognosis. Dr. Ye, very clearly described the process of an epidemic's onset, development, and complications. For example, with Disseminated Intravenous Coagulation (DIC), the most important treatment principle is cooling the blood, moving the blood, anti-thrombus, and improving capillary blood circulation. Even by today's standard, this theory is still very advanced, especially for critical cases of epidemics like COVID-19.

Xue Shengbai's *Damp-Heat Disease Chapter* systematically recorded damp-heat disease manifestations, characteristics of pulse and tongue in detail, and treatment formulas. It wasn't until Wu JuTong, who officially created Three Jiao syndrome differentiation and treatment system, that it was discovered that Warm plague caused by damp-heat always starts in the upper Jiao Lung, then middle jiao Spleen and Stomach, then lower jiao Liver and Kidney. He created a lot of formulas correspondingly. His book *Detailed analysis on febrile diseases* became one of the most remarkable documents of the Wen Bing School also because of his most popular formulas like Yin Qiao San, Sang Ju Yin, Qing Ying Tang, Xi Jiao Di Huang Tang Etc.

Until then, TCM Epidemiology tended to be complete meaning that they treated cold-induced plague with Shang Han School six meridian syndrome differentiation and treatment system, while warm-induced plague with Wen Bing School Wei, Qi, Ying, Xue and Three Jiao systems, those systems became standardized tools to analyze and treat different epidemics for later generations. Wang Mengying was the first doctor who integrated Shang Han and Wen Bing Schools theories, using Shang Han theory as longitude, Wen Bing theory as latitude, he wrote *Longitude and Latitude of Febrile diseases*, it contributed greatly to TCM especially for plagues. Doctors in later generations all followed his laws, called cold and warm in one theory.

From the Ming and Qing Dynasties, medical science in Europe which has been called Western Medicine in China was increasing in China, religious missionaries brought the knowledge into China. After bacteria was discovered, antibiotics' invention like sulfas and penicillin, and vaccine applications, more was known about plagues. Diseases like dysentery, tuberculosis, and smallpox had disturbed human beings for thousands of years, and are now totally under control. They have become treatable and curable. Western Medicine has spread all over China, people believe blindly and optimistically that all problems are resolved.

Over time, we suddenly found that the frequency of epidemics remains unchanged and even increased worldwide. New diseases, especially ones from viruses keep coming. On the other hand, problems like side effects and drug-resistance are appearing. Traditional Chinese Medicine, as a well-accepted medicine, with its wide natural resources, less side effects, and perfect efficacy, has made great contributions in the past thousands years. It has been used with Western Medicine and is called the Combination of Chinese Medicine and Western Medicine for more than a hundred years. A movement called Modernization of Traditional Chinese Medicine has been going on for the last sixty years in China with many achievements. One of those is the capillary blood circulation theory. In 1983, Professor Xiu Rijuan discovered in her research that a capillary blood circulation disturbance existed profusely in a series of infectious diseases like Epidemic Hemorrhagic Fever, Meningitis, Encephalitis etc when they become critical. Anisodamine (654-2), an active ingredient extracted from Chinese Herbal Medicine Yang Jin Hua (Datura Flower) can significantly improve blood flow perfusion by inhibiting platelets from gathering and relax spasms of the blood vessels. After extended use of her method, epidemic mortality due to inner organs function failure and acute circulatory shock decreased dramatically.

In an over half-century process of TCM modernization, thousands of Traditional Chinese Herbal Medicine active ingredients have been extracted by modern techniques, and have been tested by

Laboratory pharmaceutical researchers and formulas have been made into modern preparation like injection; many have anti-viral, antibacterial and anti-toxicity properties, they are applied in clinic for infection or epidemics effectively for diseases like H1N1, SARS, and COVID-19.

The most representative one is Artemisinin injection by Dr. Tu Youyou. Since1965, she has worked at the Chinese Academy of Traditional Chinese Medicine. After years of studying ancient TCM documents, extracting active ingredients, and successfully developing Artemisinin injection from sweet wormwood (the only effective anti-malaria drug after Quinine which was from plant too) she won the 2015 Nobel Prize in Physiology or Medicine for her discoveries concerning a novel therapy against Malaria. At the ceremony in the Royal Swedish Academy of Sciences, she said this is a gift from Traditional Chinese Medicine to all the world. People believe that is a mark of recognizing TCM's value as wisdom of thousands of years of practice.

Star anise seeds have been used in Chinese medicine for thousands of years, and contain ingredients that might have activity against bacteria, yeast, and fungi. People try star anise for treating flu like H1N1, COVID-19 because it is a good source of shikimic acid, which is used in the manufacture of oseltamivir (Tamiflu), a flu treatment, regarded as the only effective western medicine for various kinds of flu.

It is worth noting that these are standardized laws discovered in thousands of years of clinic practice. Whether a doctor used the six-meridian system, the 4 levels, or the Three Jiao System all of these were based on an epidemic's etiology, pathogenesis. These are all tools used to analyze cases of infectious diseases and to identify pathological factors through pattern differentiation. Sometimes they would combine disease diagnosis and syndrome differentiation, then apply treatment accordingly. In many cases they would use the same formula to treat different kinds of infections.

Approved by thousands of years of unremitting clinical practice, with great number of examples, practiced on a huge scale, on human beings some formulas are considered as classic or experienced formulas These are the most reliable evidence-based logical reasons that TCM can be applied for use in modern epidemics since TCM figured out the common patterns of plagues and the effective treatment formulas.

The basic understanding of Epidemics by TCM

All generations of Chinese medicine practitioners have been unremittingly exploring the epidemiological characteristics of the plague and coping methods, formed a set of systematic knowledge, can be summarized as follows:

1. Precondition of plague onset

Traditional Chinese Medicine realized at a very early time that the onset of plague relates with natural factors as preconditions, as early as the Han Dynasty, Yellow Emperor's Inner Classic has said Heaven and Earth generate plagues.

(1) Weather abnormality: This is the most important factor by TCM. Zhang Zhongjing said that seasonal pestilence plagues often happen when Spring should be warm but it's cool, or during Summer the weather should be warm but it's cold, Autumn should be cool but it's hot. *Treatise on Shang Han.*

(2) Geographic factors: In general, Cold-induced plagues are far less common than Warm-induced plague, therefore in southern China, especially the subtropical zone, plagues happen much more often. During the Ming Dynasty Zhang Jinyue described that there is toxic qi among the mountains and water in the deep southern area. Businessmen, travelers, even officers travel there actually at high risk, he wrote in *Jingyue Comprehensive books.*

(3) Social conflicts: Wars, population migration are very important factors. There must be a warm plague after an inauspicious year (war, famine) said Li Er in the *Dao De Jing*, and Zhang Jingyue found that eight or nine out of ten people contacted with plague are travelers. He mentioned this in his book *Jingyue Comprehensive books.* He also added that a person's weak

constitution is always the inner reason. "Miasma plague is contagious often when overexertion or hunger".

(4) TCM discovered Intermediate hosts, it was the first to be recorded and the earliest in medical science history. Plagues may not only transmit from person to person, but also animal to person, even plants to person (unproven). Many animals are intermediate hosts, and studies have shown that 60-70% of epidemics are common diseases between Human beings and animals, this process is called Zoonosis. *The Yellow Emperor's Inner Classic* said "Plague could not exist and be spread without being hosted by a scaled or shelled creature in the river and sea, by plume and wing insects or beast, bloody jaundice always arrives by a contagious one either in water or on earth". It clearly pointed out that animals are the intermediate hosts of plagues.

Traditionally in TCM, there are animal miasmas like bird's miasma, duck miasma, goose miasma, hornet Miasma, even pets like peacock miasma.

Zhang Zhongjing said that if domestic fowl die by themselves, it is most likely due to plagues, and they become poisonous, so do not eat them. And, he warned not to eat wild cats (SARS Intermediate hosts), or fruits that fall on ground after being bitten by insects or ants because of poison. In the *Synopsis Prescriptions Of Golden Chamber*, Li Shizheng directly warned people not to eat bats (COVD-19 Intermediate hosts) in his *Compendium of Materia Medica* from the Ming Dynasty, and he advocated eliminating rats, mosquitoes and flies. Later, he became famous for his writings in the Eliminate Four Pests Movement nationwide at the end of 1957 in China.

It has long been known that mosquitoes are important intermediate hosts. As early as the Han dynasty they were using mosquito nets.

(6) Route of plague transmission: TCM realized very early that one could get plagues from food through the mouth, from the air through breathing, through body contact, or sexual transmission.

Dr. Wu, Youke (Qin Dynasty) said: "Evil Qi enters the body through the mouth and nose smoothly while breathing". And Dr. Yuchang (Qin

Dynasty) also said: "Dirty Evil Qi easily transfers from one to another by living in the same house and sleeping together".

(7) Epidemic Characteristics: In *Discussing Writing and Explaining Characters* from the Han Dynasty an ancient Chinese dictionary explained: "Plague means everybody gets sick. The *Yellow Emperor's Inner Classic* explained further "when plagues come, everybody gets it from each other, no matter what age, and will be similar in the manifestations. Dr. Wu Jutong said "every family is the same. "An entire country is almost the same", Dr.Yu, Shiyu, Qing Dynasty.

"One year an epidemic may be relatively minor with a low mortality (1-2/10 mortality rate), another year can have an epidemic, even a pandemic with (1-2/10 survival rate)" said Dr.Yu Shiyu, Qing Dynasty. "No matter whether near or far, many people die suddenly" said the "*Yellow Emperor's Inner Classic*. Self-limiting phenomena have been discovered, like "Cold plague (Flu) will be self-cured in seven days, no more than fourteen days", *Shang Han Lun*.

"Immunization after plagues was also being observed" wrote Bao Pu Zi in *The Master of Preserving Simplicity*. Ge Hong in the Jin Dynasty said, "Don't worry about getting sick again after a plague". Dr. Zhang Jingyue (Ming Dynasty) wrote "Native and people who are from outside but live in the same area for a long time, will avoid plague like native one (This is similar to the Herd Immunity in Western medicine).

(8) Addressed the importance of Isolation and Sterilization: As early as the Shang Dynasty (1250 BC), there has been the concept of isolation which was administered by health officer, in the *Yellow Emperor's Inner Classic* it mentioned that doctors should hold their breath and then go into the plague room, it further pointed out to that in order to prevent contact and avoid evil qi, structures for plague patients should be built to keep them isolated. It also suggested building field hospitals or utilizing large mansions which were sitting empty.

City lockdowns and limiting domestic and interstate travel were suggested by famous doctors like Zhang Jingyue (Ming Dynasty). It was recommended that family members quarantine for three months, they were warned not to approach sick people, not approach the dead, not to share food from patients, or clothes from the dead. When visiting sick people, doctors would see patients back-to-back, keep a safe distance, hold their breath and not speak too much. Additionally, doctors were advised to never stay and sleep at a patient's house, no matter how far they had to travel. Sterilization by cooking or steaming was mentioned as early as Li Shizheng in the Ming Dynasty, He advocated that people boil city water to drink, officials in the Qing Dynasty already required steaming patient's clothes to prevent spreading of plague, much earlier than the invention of pasteurization in Europe (1864AC). Alcohol's importance for plague has been advised. The classic method was created as early as Xia Dynasty (2070-1600BC) in China, and it has been used as disinfectant, anti-sepsis, anesthetic and in cardiac since then. In the Chinese pictogram for medicine 醫 the upper part is a standing caped doctor operating on a patient who was injured by an arrow, by taking the arrow out from their head. The lower part of the character is a pot of alcohol used for disinfection. This was recorded much earlier than Arabic Medicine's record of alcohol disinfection. (Avicenna, 980-1037. The Canon of Medicine). Before the Shang Dynasty (1600AC-1046AC), it was popular to take herbal medicine in an alcohol solution.

Discussing writing and Explaining Characters Han Dynasty (100-121AC) said: "The doctor works by using alcohol, alcohol is for the treatment of illness.

In the Ming Dynasty Zhang Jingyue said, "alcohol can defeat plague miasma and save lives", *Comprehensive Books of Jingyue*

New Edition Of Materia Medica by Chen, Shiduo, in the Qin Dynasty summarized, "alcohol can quickly dispel all evil plagues, and prevent miasma".

(9). Government administration on plague:

The government usually did the following to manage plague:

- Appointed a health officer in charge of plague
- Created TCM doctor registration system for emergency
- Created monitoring and reporting system
- Created protocols for lockdown and travelling limitations when necessary
- Built isolation facilities to quarantine people with plague.
- Set up fire and smoke to sanitize air in town if necessary (Zhou Dynasty)
- Sanitized horse and carriage with smoke for visitors at the entrance of the city (Qin Dynasty)
- Plague officers in the customs department check for plagues like smallpox to prevent invasion from abroad (Qing Dynasty).
- Created the smallpox vaccination bureau, which spread information and techniques domestically and abroad. (Qing Dynasty).

(10). Personal ways to cope with Plagues.

During epidemics or pandemics, personal hygiene is important. TCM recommends keeping good hygiene daily. Clear the nose, eyes, mouth and throat, wash hands and shower, and only drink boiled water. All of these help to prevent infection.

Clear the nose:

When leaving the house use American Honey locust or paper to keep the nose clean. Use sesames oil in the nostrils when working with sick patients

Clear the eyes:

It is possible for contagious material to enter through eyes for some plagues. For those, use herbal eye drops which contain realgar, cinnabar, mirabilite, it helps to prevent infection.

Clear the mouth and throat:

For people who must leave their home during an epidemic, TCM suggested drinking liquor and to rinse their throat before leaving the house, and wash their mouth with toothpaste containing green tea, salt, willow twig, Once they get back home, they should drink sophorae root and rinse with alcohol. Early toothbrushes were mostly made with metal, bones and bamboo, the earliest unearthed one in China dates back to the Qin Dynasty's bronze toothbrush (BC221-206). There were more than 10 toothpaste formulas in the Northern Song Dynasty (AC960-1127) already.

Shower and skin care:

During an epidemic, taking a shower daily with herbal lotion is recommended, the lotion formulas often include Peach twig and leaf which contains Salicylic acid, a food preservative, an anti-inflammatory, a bactericide, and an antiseptic. Also, Dahurica root, a natural anti-inflammatory, anti-fungal herb, and Cypress Leaf, another anti-inflammatory, a bactericide, and an antiseptic, together called Seasonal plague shower lotion formula. It was also recommended to use natural shampoo made of Honey locust, a natural surfactant. After showering, use an herbal powder to keep the skin dry with an aroma. The formula usually is powdered rice, angelica root, pearl, honey locust etc.

China has a long tradition of recommending showers. In the Han Dynasty the law stipulated those officers must take a shower at least every five days, and wash their hair at least every three days. During the Han Dynasty, Emperor Xiao Gang 503-551AD himself wrote a book called the shower classic and advocated showers, even though there was a shower holiday for officers.

Soap and Hand body wash:

In ancient China, people used alkaloid earth, plant ash and wheat powder mixed with pig fat to make the earliest soap called Zao Dou to wash hands, as a body wash, for shower and laundry, the *Zhou Regulation. Inner Family Stipulation* said, "people must wash and clean your uniform and clothes with ash when it becomes dirty". During the Wei and Jin Period

(220-589AD), they started to add natural surfactant honey locust Zao Jiao with pig fat to make soap.

Cloth laundry and steamed:

Patient's clothes must be washed and steamed, and then others in the same family will not get sick, as mentioned in *Song Feng talking about plagues* by Liu Songfeng in the Qin Dynasty.

Food and drinking hygiene:

In the very early time, TCM realized accurately that food and drinking can be contaminated which may cause plagues. Dr. Ge Hong (283AD-343AD) said in his book *A Handbook of Formulas for Emergencies* "Generally Cholera-like diarrhea and vomiting plagues mostly come from contaminated food and fluids". So, throw away the food if there was contact with rodents, do not eat uncooked food, decayed food and raw fish. Realizing that animals can be an intermediate host of plagues, they created bans to forbid eating wild animals like wild cats and bats. *Yellow Emperor Inner Classic* said "Plague could not exist and spread without being hosted by scale or shelled creatures in rivers and seas, by plume and winged insects or beasts. Bloody jaundice always arrives from a contagious one either in water or on earth. Zhang Zhongjing said that if domestic fowl die by themselves, it is most likely due to plagues, then they become poisonous, so do not eat. And he warned not to eat wild cats (SARS Intermediate hosts), fruits that fall on ground after being bitten by insects and ants, because of poison. *Synopsis Prescriptions Of Golden Chamber*. Li Shizheng directly warned people not to eat bats (COVD-19 Intermediate hosts) in his *Compendium of Materia Medica* during the Ming Dynasty, and advocated eliminating rats, mosquitoes and flies. Water hygiene is just as important, Water contamination is often a precondition for plagues. Li Shizheng recommended only to take water from running water in the middle part of the river or lake, or water from deep ground wells. The best water source is filtered water or boiled.

Air sterilization

Fumigating a room is often an effective way to prevent and stop the spreading of plagues. Usually, the formulas in steam decoction devices include sweet worm grass, acorus gramineus soland, rhizome atractylodis, frankincense, myrrh, vinegar, or just burn a moxibustion stick to smoke the room. Modern pharmaceutical research has shown anti-viral, antibacterial, and antiseptic effects of those herbs; it was also proven from clinical application on COVID-19 in Wu Han, China.

There is a long history of those practices in China and Asia, especially during epidemics or the beginning of a new year. During a traditional festival of the dead every April, along with praying for protection from ancestors and loved ones who have passed, there are hygiene habits like emptying houses and cleaning them, eliminating the four pests (rat, mosquito, fly and flea), preventing plague by smudging with sweet worm grass and acorus gramineus soland, and drinking liquor which contains realgar for it antibiotic properties.

Medicine to prevent plagues

The *Yellow Emperor's Inner Classic* has laid the principles of plague prevention, that is to keep good vital qi inside the body and avoid toxic qi from outside. There are two kinds of formulas for this purpose. First, are formulas for emergencies for people at higher risk because of living/working in a high risk area and/or the risk of infecting family members. Small golden powder (Xiao Jing Dan, from the *Yellow Emperor's Classic*) and Over Miasma Powder (Du Zang San, by Dr. Ge Hong), are both antibiotic and antiseptic like formulas. Other formulas focus on supplementing immunity by stimulating the body to produce immune factors like Interferon. Jade Windscreen Powder (Yu Ping Feng San) accomplishes this. These are traditional formulas which have protected the Chinese Nation effectively for thousands of years.

Calm down and Meditation

To save energy, it is important for people to calm down and do meditation, practice energy exercises like Qi Gong, Ba Jing Duan, Yoga etc. The *Yellow Emperor's Inner Classic* clearly said prevention is first. The doctor should not only focus on treatment but focus even more on prevention. Doctors should emphasize the seasonal regulation of plagues, encourage patients to stay home in the winter to preserve their energy for coming spring plagues; more importantly, be completely free from wishes, ambitions and distracting thought, indifferent to fame and gain, the True energy (Zhen Qi) will come in the wake of it. When one concentrates his spirit internally and keeps a sound mind, how can any illness occur? These practices have been in place in China for millenia and have been proven to help people deal with the anxiety that accompanies epidemics and pandemics.

Earliest Antiserum Therapy and Earliest Vaccine: Variolation

In light of the philosophy that evil qi and vital qi can transform into each other, TCM discovered that too much vital qi can become evil fire, and excessive fire will eliminate vital qi. On the other hand, a minor evil qi can generate vital qi through stimulating the human body. These theories give rise directly to the creation of the earliest antiserum therapy and earliest vaccine in China called variolation. This pioneered modern immunotherapy, a revolution of medical science in epidemic diseases prevention and treatment.

Antiserum is a medicine prepared from human or animal sources containing antibodies, specific for combating an infectious disease while a vaccine is a substance usually a live or attenuated live virus itself given to stimulate the body's production of antibodies and provide immunity against a disease. Vaccines are prepared from agents like viruses, bacteria etc. that cause the disease, or a synthetic substitute. These offer the most reliable chance of prevention and treatment of epidemic diseases nowadays worldwide including COVID-19.

Dating back to the Jin Dynasty, Dr. Ge Hong (283 AD-343 AD), in his book *A Handbook of Formulas for Emergencies* he recorded emergency formulas for people bitten by rabid dogs by applying the rabid dog's brain tissue on the wound to prevent rabies infection. The theory being that this application will either prevent rabies infection, or the patient would only experience mild illness. That is the earliest extant document of TCM and earliest in medical science regarding the use of antiserums. Over a thousand years later, Louis Pasteur (1822-1895), a great French scientist, considered the Father of Microbiology, refined rabies antiserum from rabies dog's brain and spinal cord, and created the first vaccines for rabies, in the end, a remarkable breakthrough in prevention of diseases, his discoveries have saved many lives since then.

In 1901, Emil Von Behring won the first Nobel Medical Prize in history for his antiserum against diphtheria with great success. He accomplished this with assistance from the Japanese scientist Shibasaburo Kitasato who had a strong background in TCM theory and applied the concept of evil-on-evil treatment.

Dr. Ge Hong also recorded the use of honey to localize smallpox pustules. Later Medical documents recorded the use of milk to wash skin lesions of smallpox.

Royal physician Dr. Cao Yuanfang (550-630AC), Sui Dynasty, known for his aetiology and pathogenesis studies, created formulas by using powdered red spiders like baby chiggers which we know later 1910) easily carry the Rickett's organism. He treated Tsutsugamushi disease in his book *All disease's causes and manifestations*.

Furthermore, during the same period, The *Dun Huang Medical Document*, discovered in the desert of Northwest China in 1900, the book clearly recorded using rabbit skin for green bean sores. It advised using rabbit skin first, and later rabbit meat or fur (in England they used wool). Most likely rabbits and sheep were infected with cowpox (vaccinia), so these products were used for prevention and treatment of human smallpox, which were called green bean sores back then.

It was during the Tang Dynasty Kai (713-741AD), 400 years after smallpox spread into China due to the war with the Huns (283AD), that millions of people and soldiers died. Dr. Zhao from southern China started teaching and applying inoculation techniques called Bi Miao鼻苗. This literally translates as planting a sprout inside the nose after bloodletting, actually using dried scab powder from recovered smallpox patients. That is the first primary vaccine variation used in clinics and then recorded in books on variolation. This was recorded in the Qing Dynasty by Dong Yushan in the *New Vaccinia Book*.

Variolation was very successful since the Song Dynasty and after the Tang dynasty, most of the smallpox patients were children. They even regarded smallpox as a children's disease and information was recorded in Pediatrics books; adults seemed to be immune. In the book of successful cases called the *Concluded Smallpox Compendium* was a young boy called Wang Su, son of Wang Dan, a famous Prime Minister. He was saddened because a few of his children died from smallpox. Wang Dan decided to invite a priest, Qing Feng, by offering him big money. The priest came to the capitol from Sichuan, a long distance. Qing Feng who enjoyed a good reputation for variolation then (success rate >90%) managed to reduce Wang Su's fever and rash within three days, very gently, and the child totally recovered in twelve days and was immunized for his entire life. Wang Su died at the age of 67 years old.

In the Ming Dynasty, the greatest pharmacologist in TCM history Li Shizhen (1518-1593AD) in his great pharmacopoeia book recorded that boophilus, a kind of tick that sucks the blood from cattle, is a very common intermediate host of epidemics. As a medicine, its main action is to prevent smallpox, it is taken after being baked and powdered. A significant challenge in the Qing Dynasty was for Manchurians who had never been exposed to smallpox from generation to generation. After conquering part of China, they immigrated from far the northern area beyond the great wall as nomads. There they encountered the disaster of smallpox and many people died. Four emperors from the twelve Qing Dynasty Emperors were infected, two of them died sequentially. Emperor Kang Xi who suffered from smallpox and survived with disfigurement on his face, ordered the construction of a secondary palace to escape smallpox. He hired the royal variolation doctor, Zhu Cungu was the first one, he appointed a national variolation officer who oversaw inoculation in China and dependent states. He instituted a quarantine for foreigners and businessmen who had business in foreign countries, he built schools and smallpox hospitals, he issued mandatory laws for variolation application inside China and dependent states. He certified citizens after inoculation and ordered people who were not inoculated to stay home. They were not allowed to go out during the epidemic, and officers were not allowed to have an audience with the Emperor.

TCM has been called the primary seed for modern vaccines until now this means like a seed sprout, after being planted or inoculated in the body, the vital qi, once stimulated, will flourish and fight evil plagues. Traditionally, there were four kinds of variolation methods:

(1). Pox clothes method: The healthy person would wear the inner layer of an infected patient›s clothes of a patient who is suffering from smallpox in order to get infected and become immunized from plague. This method was not popular because the success rate was low, the risk level was low as well

(2). Pox liquid method: They would collect the thick liquid from the scabs of smallpox patients, apply it to the nostril of a healthy person after pricking the membrane. This method had a higher success rate and higher risk too.

(3). Dried sprout method: They would take fine, powdered scabs from smallpox patients, blow the powder into the nostril of a healthy person. This method was successful but uncomfortable.

(4). Watery sprout method: They would prepare a decoction of fine scab powder mixed with clean water or milk, apply it into the nostril with a cotton ball, and keep it for 12 hours. This method had a good success rate, it was safe, easy to perform, and was the most popular one in ancient times.

There were two kinds of Sprout Methods for variolation: Fresh Sprout and Matured Sprout. The Fresh Sprout Method used a scab that was collected for the first time from a smallpox patient, this method offered more side effects and was considered high risk. The best method was the so-called Matured Sprout Method, which took the scab from a healthy, inoculated person and passed it from one to another safely again and again. The longer the time the better. There were very little or no side effects, the action was much gentler and the success rate was much higher.

Choosing seed sprouts required skill and care in order to get the best results. A few measures have to be followed in order to produce a seed sprout culture that would enter the body.

(1). Choose matured sprouts as much as possible and use them as much as possible (Attenuated vaccine).

(2). Ideally, sprouts were chosen from a successive case that had minimal side effects.

(3). The scabs should look like wax, being pale and bright. They should not be dark, bleeding, smelly, thick, fatty, or large.

(4). Seed sprouts had to be processed to reduce toxicity (attenuated). This was done by drying them and grinding them into a fine powder. They were stored in glass bottles and buried underground.

(5). Sprouts were diluted with clear water or human milk before use.

The book *Variolation Heartfelt Methods,* during the Qing Dynasty summarized: The seed sprout that was used for a longer time contains a purer action as a medicine. Being more mature, the evil fire toxin decreased over time, yet the vital essence still exists, therefore being harmless and guaranteed.

Variolation practitioners kept matured sprouts in glass bottles underground where temperatures were colder and used them in their variolation clinic as a family business. Some for hundreds of years. The best branch was from southern China called the Tai Ping Sprout (Peaceful sprout, meaning the safest one), and these were used for a long time.

Variolation methods improved so much that the government would not accept a failure rate higher than 5% in the later Qing Dynasty. Emperor Kang Xi performed a successful trial on his own children, then the children of aristocrats, then promoted variolation across all of China. According to records, millions of lives were saved.

The variolation method then spread all over the world. In 1688, the Russian government sent international students to learn variolation in Beijing, and then the method spread to Russia. In 1744, the Chinese doctor Li Renshan introduced variolation in Nagasaki, Japan.

In 1790, the Korean messenger Piao Zaijia brought TCM books back to Korea including *Children variolation Heartfelt method* from China. In 1721, Lady Mary Wortley Montagu, the wife of the British ambassador to Turkey, performed variolation on her son, then her daughter in Istanbul, then she introduced it to England, after successful tests were performed on prisoners. The Queen mandated variolation in England, then the method spread to all of Europe, India and even North America.

Enlightened by the TCM variolation method, British countryside doctors also practiced variolation. Edward Jenner (1749-1823) created the cowpox vaccine in 1798. He discovered that women who worked on cattle farms obtained lifetime immunity from smallpox after being infected with cowpox, a virus very similar to human smallpox which can infect animals like cows, sheep, rabbits and humans. Cowpox vaccine is much more effective and much safer, soon it became popular all over the world, including China, it marked the beginning of modern immunology.

After the cowpox vaccine, scientists developed many vaccines that are effective against epidemic diseases. Many of these epidemic diseases have become treatable and controllable. In 1980, the WHO announced smallpox eradication.

It is widely considered true that TCM variolation is the pioneer of vaccination. It was highly valued by the French enlightenment writer and philosopher Voltaire, he said "I have heard that the Chinese kept this for a hundred years.

COVID-19 is the worst disease in recent centuries. There are already vaccines developed in America, Europe, India, China and Russia with high effectiveness rates (50-96%). Pfizer, Moderna, Sanofi, Johnson, and Johnson etc, and antiserum therapy have shown very desirable results in initial studies, conclusions cannot be confirmed on their safety and side effects. New strains and variants of COVID-19 like B1.617, B117, P1 keep coming causing subsequent waves requiring more doses of vaccine, perhaps requiring annual inoculation. Vaccine is the most hopeful method to prevent further spread of COVID-19.

The monoclonal antibody treatment bamlanivimab has been given emergency use authorization by the US Food and Drug Administration for treating mild to moderate covid-19 in adults and children who have not been admitted to a hospital.

The FDA says that bamlanivimab has been shown to reduce covid-19 related hospital admission or emergency room visits in patients at high risk for disease progression in the 28 days after treatment when compared with placebo. Bamlanivimab acts against the SARS-CoV-2 spike protein to stop the virus attaching to and entering human cells; it has become the most hopeful drug in the future to treat COVID-19.

Some poisonous plant-sourced medicines have shown an inspiring result, like Quinine which is derived from Cinchona tree in South America for malaria. Chloroquine and hydroxychloroquine have been found to be efficient on SARS-CoV-2 and reported to be efficient in Chinese COV-19 patients. A trial evaluating the role of hydroxychloroquine on respiratory viral loads has been done in France. Patients were included in a single arm protocol to receive 600mg of hydroxychloroquine daily and their viral load in nasal swabs was tested daily. Depending on their clinical presentation, azithromycin was added to the treatment. Untreated patients from another center and cases refusing the protocol were included as negative controls. Presence and absence of virus at Day6-post inclusion was considered the end point. Results showed 20 cases were treated in this study and showed a significant reduction of the viral carriage at D6-post inclusion compared to controls, and much lower average carrying duration than reported of untreated patients in the literature. Azithromycin added to hydroxychloroquine was significantly more efficient for virus elimination. Conclusion is that Hydroxychloroquine is significantly associated with viral load reduction/disappearance in COVID-19 patients and its effect is reinforced by azithromycin. This clinical trial was approved by the French National Agency for Drug safety (ANSM) (2020-000890-25) and to the French Ethic Committee (CPP Ile de France) (20.02.28.99113) for reviewing and approved on 5th and 6th March, 2020, respectively. This trial is registered with EU Clinical trials register number 2020-000890-25.

Colchicine from wild lily which is a TCM herbal medicine for cough. The Montreal Heart Institute (MHI) has announced positive, clinically persuasive results from the COLCORONA clinical trial of the orally administered drug, colchicine, for treating Covid-19. The contact-less, randomized, double-blind, placebo-controlled clinical trial was conducted in an at-home setting in Canada, US, Europe, South America and South Africa. It analyzed whether colchicine could lower the risk of severe complications linked to Covid-19. There were approximately 4,500 Covid-19 patients who were not hospitalized at the time of enrolment and had a minimum of one risk factor for Covid-19 complications. According to the study, results obtained from 4,488 patients, colchicine lowered the risk of death or hospitalizations by 21% in Covid-19 patients versus placebo, approaching statistical significance. Furthermore, the analysis of the 4,159 Covid-19 patients receiving colchicine showed statistically significant reductions in the risk of death or hospitalization versus placebo. In these Covid-19 patients, the drug lowered hospitalizations by 25%, the requirement for mechanical ventilation by 50% and deaths by 44%. The Institute noted that the latest scientific discovery makes colchicine the world's first oral drug which can be used for treating non-hospitalized Covid-19 patients, but still there is no special approved safe drug for COVID-19. For this, it is necessary to overview how TCM treats epidemic diseases by different schools in history, mainly Shang Han School which mostly treated for cold induced plagues, and the Wen Bing School which mostly treated for warmth induced plagues.

The Schools of TCM on Plague Understanding and Treatment

Plagues can be divided into two categories in TCM: Cold-induced and Warm-induced, correspondingly by the diagnosis, differentiation, and treatment. Two major schools were formed, the school which focused on cold-induced disorders, called the Shang Han School, and the school which focused on warm-induced disorder, called the Wen Bing School.

Shang Han School Theory: Six Meridian syndrome differentiation and Treatment System

The Shang Han school founded by Dr. Zhang Zhongjing, Eastern Han Dynasty (150-219 A.D), he was the author of the classic Chinese text *Treatise on Febrile diseases and miscellaneous diseases* (Shan Han Za Bing Lun) 伤寒杂病论. We believe that this is the first extant medical book on infectious and epidemic diseases, especially influenza. The reasons are the following:

1. Shang Han (in Chinese it means exogenous cold-induced disease) was defined as a febrile disease by the NanJing *Medical difficulty Questions*. It is a sort of infectious disease, Zhang Zhongjing followed up on the laws of the Nan Jing and Nei Jing *Yellow Emperor Inner Classic* academically which he claimed in the preface of his book.

2. Shang Han refers to groups of contagious epidemics. Zhang Zhongjing said in the preface of his book, 2/3 people from 200 in his patriarchal clan died within ten years, seven out of ten were due to Shang Han.

3. Shang Han diseases are related to winter and cold weather or climatic abnormalities during flu season, typically happening annually.

4. Shang Han diseases manifest as upper respiratory infections like influenza. Symptoms and signs include fever, chills, headache, body aches, sneezing, nose running, cough, wheezing. vomiting and diarrhea.

5. Incubation period: 1-7days.
6. Natural duration is 7-13 days.
7. There is a self-limiting trend.
8. Frequent complications include bronchitis, pneumonia, asthma, sometimes pericarditis, myocarditis etc.
9. All of the above-mentioned match in etiology, pathology, symptoms and signs with upper respiratory infection like influenza.
10. There is a chapter on Cholera-like acute gastroenteritis (likely due to Stomach Flu) and dysentery etc. including other infectious diseases.
11. Epidemic hemorrhagic fever may be part of the Shang Han group since Kidney failure (Tai Yang blood retention), but most likely to be Yin Yang Toxin in Golden Cabinet (Jin Gui Yao Lue).
12. Although the plague and smallpox started as epidemics in China during the Han dynasty, neither are self-limiting, their natural durations are much longer, and the prognosis is much worse. In the Ming Dynasty, doctors recorded that formulas from the *Shang Han Lun did not* work for Smallpox, so Shang Han in the *Shang Han Lun* most likely are not referring to smallpox and the plague.

Dr. Zhang Zhongjing discovered that cold-induced plagues which he called Shang Han mostly start with one of the three yang stages, then move to the three yin stages. Yang stages which are in the upper respiratory system last about 7-14 days and prognosis is good. And they most likely will be self-limiting. If the situation gets worse instead of getting better, the disease will go deeper into the interior to the three yin stages located in the lower respiratory system. Commonly, Lung infection (Tai Yin) will be involved. Heart, Liver and brain damage may show (Jue Yin) in severe cases, and deadly Heart failure or Kidney damage (Shao Yin) may happen in the critical stages.

Shang Han disease may start with a combination of Yang and Yin stages like Tai Yang/Tai Yin symptoms simultaneously. For example, in the case of Stomach flu. The severity of the disease will depend on the strength of the primary disease and the constitution of the patient. The pathogen may enter at a superficial Yang stage, but rapidly invade the interior causing a critical situation with a poor prognosis.

Initially in the superficial Tai Yang stage symptoms manifest as fever, chills. Then it may enter the Shao Yang stage, which lies between the exterior and the interior manifesting symptoms like alternating fever and chills. The disease may resolve at this point or enter the interior Yang Ming stage with high fever, thirst, red face, and sweating. The three yang stages will not last for a long time, many less than 2 weeks and many will be self-limiting. Or patients will be cured by treatment in the clinic. This is the most common outcome.

The three Yin stages are seen less often in the TCM clinic these days. Although we can assume that they were encountered more often in Zhang Zhongjing's time, much earlier than the first antibiotic invented in 1929. Tai Yin stages mainly manifest as cough and wheezing related to acute bronchitis, pneumonia, even Lung abscess. If the disease progresses many complications appear due to septicemia like Pericarditis, Myocarditis, brain damage, manifesting as convulsions, unconsciousness (Jue Ying stage related to Pericardium and Liver), and life-threatening toxic shock. Heart failure or renal failure may happen in the end, this is called Shao Ying stage relating to Heart and Kidney. After understanding Shang Han's general patterns, Zhang Zhongjing created formulas and applied those formulas at his busy clinic accordingly. These formulas are so effective that later generations called them classic formulas or experienced formulas. They have been applied very effectively for influenza or influenza-like epidemic diseases including SARS and COVID-19. He systematically studied Shang Han disease's onset, development and treatment; he formed the Shang Han School. Shang Han Lun became the most important standard theory to understand and treat epidemic diseases. It has been collected and kept as a strategic book by Emperors' governments, later spreading to Japan, Korea, Vietnam and all over Northern, Eastern, and SouthEast Asia.

We can summarize the Shang Han Syndrome differentiation and Treatment theory as following:

(The dosage for each herb in formulas is from the writer's personal experience).

Taiyang Syndrome

Symptoms and signs: Stiff neck, headache, fever, aversion to cold, floating pulse

- For people with weak constitution, Wind cold exterior deficiency: Gui zhi tang.
- For people with strong constitution, Wind cold exterior excesses: Ma huang tang.

Gui Zhi Tang (Cinnamon Decoction)

Gui Zhi	Ramulus Cinnamomi	15g
Bai Shao	Paeonia Lactiflora	12g
Shen Jiang	Zingiber Officinale	12g
Da Zao	Ziziphus Jujuba Mill	9g
Zhi Gan	Cao Glycyrrhiza Uralensis	6g

Ma Huang tang	(Ephedra decoction)	
Ma Huang	Ephedrae	6g
Gui Zhi	Ramulus Cinnamomi	12g
Xing Ren	Semen Armeniacae Amarum	12g
Zhi Gan Cao	Glycyrrhiza Uralensis	6g

Comment:

All doses above herbs should be adjusted by practitioners according to differentiation (the following are the same). The Tai Yang stage is the initial period like the sun appearing in the early morning (Tai Yang literally means the sun). The patient shows aversion to wind and cold, with goose bumps, headache, body pain. Ma Huang, Gui Zhi, Sheng Jiang are warm, pungent, and acrid in nature. They can release the exterior wind-cold. Modern pharmaceutical research has shown these herbs have a reliable wide spectrum inhibitory effect on influenza A, B, Coronavirus, Rhinovirus etc. These herbs have also shown a diaphoretic effect to lower temperature as well as an analgesic effect. They can improve a patient's general condition, much earlier than the first diaphoretics like Aspirin which is also naturally sourced from white willow bark. For people with poor constitution, overuse of diaphoretics is harmful, therefore there is only Gui Zhi without Ma Huang in Gui Zhi Tang.

Xing Ren can dilute phlegm and relieve cough, while honey cooked Gan Cao is not only like steroids in chemical structure, but also like steroids in their anti-inflammatory function.

Gui Zhi Tang and Ma Huang Tang are still the most popular formulas for influenza or flu-like epidemic diseases.

Tai yang syndrome complications

Tai yang water retention syndrome (Acute glomerulonephritis)

Symptoms: aversion to wind, fever, difficulty in urination, extreme thirst, vomiting immediately after drinking, and floating pulse.

Wu ling san (Five Ingredients with Poria Powder)

Gui Zhi	Ramulus Cinnamomi	15g
Bai Zhu	Atractylodes Macrocephala	12g
Fu Ling	Poria	12g
Zhu Ling	Polyporus umbellatus	12g
Ze Xie	Rhizoma Alismatis	12g

Tai yang blood retention syndrome (Hemolytic Uremic Syndrome)

Symptoms: aversion to wind, fever, stiffness and fullness feeling in lower abdomen, enuresis, mental disorder, even madness, deep and thread pulse.

Tao He Cheng Qi Tang (Peach Pit Decoction to Order the Qi)

Tao Ren	Persicae Semen	15g
Gui Zhi	Ramulus Cinnamomi	12g
Da Huang	Rheum Palmatum	9g
Zhi Gan Cao	Glycyrrhiza Uralensis	6g

Comments

Renal complications of influenza virus infections are uncommon but can contribute to deterioration in the patient's condition and even death. These include acute Kidney injury (AKI), acute glomerulonephritis (AGN), disseminated intravascular coagulation (DIC), and hemolytic uremic syndrome (HUS). Dr. Zhang Zhongjing was the first person to discover those pneumonias, and named them as Tai Yang Syndrome complications, Tai Yang Water retention (AGN), Tai Yang Blood retention respectively (HUS), and created effective formulas for those. Nowadays Wu Ling san is still the most popular formula for AGN, and Tao He Cheng Qi Tang for AKI, and HUS.

Pharmacological research showed that Wu Ling San can promote urination. The volume increased 110% after using Wu Ling San, which is similar to western medicine diuretics. Wu Ling San was used in the treatment of acute glomerulonephritis, 78 cases, and edema due to nephritis, 42 cases, with an efficacy rate of 90% (China Chinese Medicine report 2020-7-6.) Xi Anquan treated acute glomerulonephritis, 38 cases, with Wu Ling san, 36 cases cured, 2 improved. Sun Jianping treated the early stage of renal functional failure, very effectively, 6 cases, and partly-effective, 8 cases, with a total efficacy rate of 70% (Xia, Liming. Clinic application and modern study on Wu Ling San. Progress in modern biomedicine. 2006 vol.6. no.6.75).

By exploring the effects of Tao He Cheng Qi Tang on microinflammation factors in rats with chronic renal failure, the mechanism of treating chronic renal failure (CRF) microinflammation of Tao He Cheng Qi Tang is clarified. Method: 60 clean male SD rats, 7 weeks old, body mass 180 to 200g, randomly divided into normal group, false surgery group, model group, control group, treatment group each with 12 rats. The model group, control group and treatment group all used the international 5/6 renal excision animal model and performed 5/6 renal excision surgery. The fake surgical group only does double Kidney membrane peeling, Blank group gets no operation. After continuous administration of 56d after surgery, the content of CRP, TNF-α, IL-6, ALB was detected by ELISA method, and the Kidney tissue was observed by electroscope to observe the ultrastructure of Kidney tissue. Results was content of CRP, TNF-α and IL-6 in Tao He Cheng Qi Tang group was significantly reduced compared with the model group and control group (P.05); Compared with the model group and the control group, the ALB content in Tao He Cheng Qi Tang group increased significantly (P.05). Conclusion: Tao He Cheng Qi Tang inhibits the increase of inflammatory factors CRP, TNF-α and IL-6, it increases the content of ALB and improves the fibrosis of CRF nephrocytes, which may be one of the mechanisms of CRF (Zhang, Xikui etc. Journal of Yunnan University of Traditional Chinese Medicine. Vol.39. No.3. 2016. Jun.) Ma Lai used 125 wistar rats in a Kidney failure model and treated with Tao He Chen Qi Tang in 5 groups. The results showed that the treatment group RBC, HB were higher than control group (P<0.05), Scr, BUN decreased (P<0.05), Kidney tissue Smad3, CTFGmRNA decreased (P<0.05), Smad7mRNA increased (P<0.05), indicated that Tao He Cheng Qi Tang can relieve symptoms of renal functional failure, correct anemia, delay Kidney unit degeneration and fibrosis. Zhao Zhongjiang et al treated 20 cases of renal functional failure with Tao He Cheng Qi Tang, relieved 4 cases, 10 very effective cases, 3 cases considered effective, with a total efficacy rate of 85%. They found that Tao He Cheng Qi Tang lowered patient's Scr, Bun, increased Hb, Rbc, improved anemia condition, and improved high coagulation condition of the Kidneys (Journal of Hebei University of Traditional Chinese Medicine. 1995.No.2).

2. Shaoyang Syndrome

Symptoms and signs: alternating chills and fever, fullness sensation in chest and hypochondria, aversion to food, vexation, vomiting, bitter taste in mouth, dry throat and dizziness.

Xiao chai hu tang (Small Thorowax Decoction)

Chai Hu	Bupleuri Radix	15g
Huang Qin	Scutellaria baicalensis Georgi	12g
Ban Xia 15	Pinellia Ternata Breit	12g
Shen Jiang 9	Zingiber Officinale	12g
Ren Shen 15	Panax ginseng	12g
Gan Cao 3	Glycyrrhiza Uralensis	6g
Da Zao 6	Ziziphus Jujuba Mill	9g

Combined syndrome of Taiyang and Shaoyang: Chai Hu Jia Gui Zhi Tang

Combined syndrome of Yangming and Shaoyang: Da Chai Hu Tang

Chai Hu Jia Gui Zhi Tang: Xiao Chai Hu Tang add Gui Zhi, Bai Shao

Da Chai Hu Tang (Big Thorowax Decoction)

Chai Hu	Bupleuri Radix	15g
Bai Shao	Paeonia Lactiflora Pall	12g
Huang Qin	Scutellaria baicalensis Georgi	12g
Ban Xia	Pinellia Ternata Breit	12g
Shen Jiang	Zingiber Officinale	12g
Da Zao	Ziziphus Jujuba Mill	9g
Da Huang	Rheum Palmatum	9g
Zhi Shi	Citrus aurantium	12g

Comments

Shao Yang means a rising sun literally, Shao Yang stage is located between the exterior and the interior. The evil qi is strong while vital qi is also strong, the struggling stalemate will determine prognosis. It may be relieved on its own as the body expels the pathogen or through initial treatment. In some cases, the patient will become worse as the pathogen moves into the interior Yang Ming stage. So, it may combine with Tai Yang syndrome, or with Yang Ming syndrome.

Xiao Chai Hu Tang works to supplement vital qi with Ren Shen while relieving Shao Yang stage with Chai Hu which is an approved antipyretic. Other symptoms like vomiting are treated with Sheng Jiang, a natural anti-emetic.

3. Yang Ming Syndrome

Symptoms: high fever, profuse spontaneous perspiration, red face, extreme thirst for drinking, aversion to heat, full and pulse, and yellow and dry coating.

Bai Hu Tang. (White Tiger Decoction)

Shi Gao	Gypsum Fibrosum	24g
Zhi Mu	Anemarrhenae Rhizoma	15g
Sticky rice	Oryza Sativa	25g
Gan Cao	Glycyrrhiza Uralensis	6g

Comments

Yang Ming literally means bright sunshine. After the Tai Yang stage and Shao Yang stage, the fight between vital qi and evil qi worsened, most likely complicated with a bacterial infection, resulting in complications like Pharyngitis, Laryngitis, Sinusitis, Otitis Media etc. Endotoxins from bacteria lead to the condition deteriorating further and manifesting as the four big symptoms: high fever, red face, sweating, thirst, and flooding pulse which Dr. Zhang Zhongjing described as Yang Ming syndrome.

Yang Ming heat can damage Qi and Yin, causing electrolyte disturbances and dehydration. Bai Hu Tang is an approved weak antibiotic, strong antipyretic, anti-inflammatory formula. Lead by Shi Gao, paired with Zhi Mu, then adding steroid-like anti-inflammatory agent Gan Cao. Rice contains sugar and electrolytes, cooked rice soup can replenish electrolytes, reverse dehydration, supplement Qi and Yin, similar to ORS (rehydration salt), it is very important during febrile disease treatment.

Complication of Yang Ming Syndrome:

As you can see in Bai Hu Tang there is a lack of strong antibiotic herbs like later generation's Huang Lian Jie Du Tang. An uncontrolled severe infection like pneumonia may cause toxic paralytic intestine obstruction which Dr. Zhang Zhongjing called Yang Ming Organ syndrome, it manifests as severe fullness sensation and pain in the abdomen, constipation, tidal fever, delirium, deep and forceful pulse. Dr. Zhang Zhongjing discovered it and named it as Yang Ming Fu syndrome, and created an effective formula: Cheng Qi tang to purge the intestines, clear heat toxins, and reactivate intestine Qi. Nowadays it is still used successfully instead of surgery.

Da Cheng Qi Tang (Major Order the Qi Decoction)

Da Huang	Rheum Palmatum	15g
Mang Xiao	Natrii Sulfas	12g
Zhi Shi	Citrus aurantium	12g
Huo Po	Magnolia Officinalis	12g

Comment:

Da Huang is a purgative which works mechanically, more importantly, it is a strong detoxifying medicine for endotoxins from bacteria, and endotoxins resulting in toxic paralytic intestine obstruction which is common in the clinic when an infection becomes uncontrollable. Da Huang is an antibiotic-like herb and an enhanced anti-inflammatory with the mineral Mang Xiao as well, together with Zhi Shi and Hou Po, it can purge the intestines better and reduce abdominal cavity pressure.

64 cases of intestinal obstruction patients had been randomly divided into observation group and control group, both groups regularly used fasting, intravenous nutritional support, gastrointestinal decompression, and maintained the balance of hydroelectric solutions. Timely use of antibiotics to fight infection, if necessary, should also use anti-spasms and painkillers to relieve the suffering of these patients. Somatostatin 3mg (Canlinin) continuous intravenous pumping for 7 days for both groups, and the observation group added Da Cheng Qi Tang by enema 100ml/ twice a day for 7 days. The result was of the 32 patients in the observation group with intestinal obstruction, 23 were cured, 7 were effective, and the total effectiveness of treatment was 93. 8%; of the 32 patients with intestinal obstruction in the control group, 18 were cured, 6 were effective, with a total treatment effective rate of 75%, and P<0.05, Da Cheng Qi Tang group had better results, indicated that Da Chen Qi Tang is effective to intestine obstruction.

4. TaiYin syndrome

Symptoms: Fullness sensation in the abdomen and vomiting, no appetite, uncontrolled worsening and watery diarrhea. Abdominal pain may present if treated incorrectly with purgative, then the hardness and fullness feeling will increase below the chest.

Tai Yin syndrome with exterior:

Gui Zhi	Ramulus Cinnamomi	15g
Bai Shao	Paeonia Lactiflora	12g
Sheng Jiang	Zingiber Officinale	12g
Da Zao	Ziziphus Jujuba Mill	9g
Zhi Gan Cao	Glycyrrhiza Uralensis	6g

Tai Yin syndrome with interior pain: Gui Zhi Jia Shao Yao Tang

Tai Yin syndrome with interior excesses: Gui Zhi Jia Da Huang Tang

Gui Zhi	Ramulus Cinnamomi	15g
Bai Shao	Paeonia Lactiflora	12g
Sheng Jiang	Zingiber Officinale	12g
Da Zao	Ziziphus Jujuba Mill	9g
Zhi Gan Cao	Glycyrrhiza Uralensis	6g
Da Huang	Rheum Palmatum	9g

Tai Yin with damp-heat in the interior and exterior: Ge Gen Huang Qin Huang Lian Tang.

Ge Gen	Pueraria Lobata (willd)	15g
Huang Qin	Scutellaria baicalensis Georgi	12g
Huang Lian	Coptis Salisb	12g
Zhi Gan Cao	Glycyrrhiza Uralensis	6g

Tai Yin damp-heat in the interior only: Xie Xin Tang (Purge and clean the Middle Decoction)

Da Huang	Rheum Palmatum	12g
Huang Qin	Scutellaria baicalensis Georgi	15g
Huang Lian	Coptis Salisb	15g
Zhi Gan Cao	Glycyrrhiza Uralensis	6g

If anuria is present (Acute prerenal functional failure) add:

Wu ling san (Five Ingredient with Poria Powder)

Gui Zhi	Ramulus Cinnamomi	15g
Bai Zhu	Atractylodes Macrocephala	12g
Fu Ling	Poria	12g
Zhu Ling	Polyporus umbellatus	12g
Ze Xie	Alisma plantago-aquatica Linn	12g

Severe uncontrolled diarrhea:

Chi Shi Zhi Yu Yu Liang Wan.

Chi Shi Zhi Halloysitum Rubrum	15g
Yu Yu Liang Limonitum	12g

Tao Hua Tang (Peach blossom decoction)

Chi Shi Zhi	Halloysitum Rubrum	15g
Gan Jiang	Zingiber Officinale	12g
Gen Mi	Oryza Sativa L	25g

With interior deficiency cold:

Li Zhong Tang (Organize Middle Jiao Decoction)

Ren Sheng	Panax ginseng C.A.Meyer	15g
Bai Zhu	Atractylodis Macrocephalae Rhizoma	12g
Gan Jiang	Zingiber Officinale	12g
Zhi Gan Cao	Glycyrrhiza Uralensis	6g

Or Si Ni Tang. (Frigid Extremities Decoction)

Fu Zi	Aconiti Lateralis Radix Praeparata	15g
Gan Jiang	Zingiber Officinale	12g
Zhi Gan Cao	Glycyrrhiza Uralensis	6g

Comments:

Stomach Flu (Viral gastroenteritis) is an intestinal infection often caused by influenza viruses like Norovirus, Rotavirus, Echo virus etc. prevalent during the autumn and winter every year, marked by watery diarrhea, abdominal cramps, nausea or vomiting, and sometimes fever. Dehydration and electrolyte disturbances are common, and infection may result in circulatory failure and even cause death. This is severe yang deficiency with Yang collapse according to TCM. It was Dr. Zhang Zhongjing who discovered this and recorded it in the *Shang Han Lun*, he created a series of effective formulas. When the disease started, Zhang Zhongjing called it a Tai Yin wind attack, and used Gui Zhi Tang to expel wind-cold, while harmonizing the interior; if there is interior heat, use Ge Gen Huang Qin Huang Lian Tang.

To observe the clinical effects of Qinlian Tongxie Granule (which is based on Ge Gen Huang Qin Huang Lian Tang) in treating acute gastroenteritis (damp-heat type) with pain and diarrhea, 400 patients were randomly divided into two groups. The control group was treated with Western medicine, the experimental group was treated with oral Qinlian Tongxie granules and returned the next day. The observed indicators of the two groups were the main curative effects (anti diarrhea) and secondary curative effects (slow pain, antiemetic, etc.). Results: the total clinical efficacy of the control group was 77.5%, and the total clinical efficiency of the experimental group was 85%. There was no statistically significant difference (P>0.05). 2) Secondary efficacy: The total clinical efficacy of the control group and the experimental group was 88.95% and 95.1% respectively, there were differences in the tests. The rate of abdominal pain and vomiting and the incidence of side effects were observed respectively. It was found that the effective rate of abdominal pain and antiemesis in the experimental group was higher than that of the control group (P<0.05), and the incidence of side effects was not statistically significant (P>0.05). [Conclusion] Qinlian Tongxie Granule is effective in treating acute gastroenteritis (damp-heat type). The effect of anti-diarrhea is similar to that of Western medicine. The antiemetic effect is superior to western medicine. It is highly safe and worthy of clinical application. (Wu Wen, Xu Boliang, Zhu Sen. Clinical observation on the treatment of acute gastroenteritis with Qinlian Tongxie Granule [J]. Journal of Tianjin University of Traditional Chinese Medicine, 2020, 39(6): 665-668.) In cases where diarrhea is so severe, use Chi Shi Zhi Yu Yu Liang Wan, which contains Kaolin clay (same active ingredient with Montmorillonite clay, the brand name is Smecta, it is a natural silicate of aluminium and magnesium used as an intestinal adsorbent in the treatment of severe gastrointestinal diseases), it is an astringent, and it can quickly stop diarrhea. If there is dehydration and electrolyte imbalance, add sticky rice and Gan Jiang to Chi Shi Zhi, this is called Tao Hua Tang (Peach flower like decoction), essentially it is a combination of rice soup together with astringent, a very advanced technique dating back to almost 2000years ago.

If the diarrhea becomes chronic, Li Zhong Tang is needed. If dehydration and electrolytes imbalance cause circulatory failure resulting in renal functional failure manifesting as enuresis, then a diuretic formula like Wu Ling San is needed (*Shang Han Lun*).

In later stages, shock, Heart failure and Kidney failure may occur. This is the Shao Yin stage. The earliest effective anti-shock agent, cardiotonic like formula Si Ni San was first written in the *Shang Han Lun*. It is still the number one rescuer for those emergency conditions nowadays in Chinese TCM hospitals injections. It is delivered as an injection.

Much of the pharmacological research on Si Ni Tang has shown that Si Ni Tang elevates blood pressure, it is cardiotonic and has an anti-shock effect. A study published in the journal Chinese Medicine Research, 1983; 2:26 uses anesthesia-induced rabbit's low blood pressure state as a model to observe Si Ni Tang and its single component's effect. The results showed that although Fu Zi has a strong cardiotonic effect, it is not as effective as Si Ni Tang, and can cause ectopic arrhythmia. The three-herb combination of Si Ni Tang cardiotonic effect is better, and can slow down the sinus Heart rate, avoid the abnormal arrhythmia caused by single Fu Zi, suggesting the rationality of the multi-ingredient formula. It also reflects the Chinese medicine saying, "Fu Zi is not hot if without Gan Jiang, Gan Cao can harmonize Fu zi ".

In the Journal of New Medicine (1974; 3:21) report it is written "It has been observed that Si Ni Tang intramuscular or intravenous injections have the following effects: (1) It improves shock status. The study reported that 20 minutes after the injection the blood pressure rose to 90-110/60-90 mmHg, up from 60-80 mmHg. Once the blood pressure reached a normal level it did not continue to rise. (2) It improves microcirculation.

For patients with cold limbs, gray lips and skin or bruising, the first step is to warm the limbs, indicating that the quality and dynamics of the blood flow perfusion may be improved in the internal organs. Heart rate generally does not decrease, but the strength is increased. The Heart tone was strong, the pulse was strong. (3) It prevents shock. Si Ni Tang injections have proved to have this effect, the cardiotonic effect is obvious.

In short, it is believed that the role of Si Ni Tang injection does not simply elevate blood pressure, but also has a cardiotonic effect and improves microcirculation, as well as offering a tranquilizing effect. "Chinese medicine research" (1985; 9:24): Si Ni Tang can prevent several animal shocks, such as caused by blood loss, hypoxic and coronary-artery-ligation. And there is a significant cardiotonic effect, it can increase the flow of blood in the coronary vessels. It can also excite the pituitary, adrenal cortex function. It has a central nervous system analgesic, sedative effect, and the toxicity is not obvious.

Tianjin Medical Newsletter (1972; 11:1): Of the 105 patients treated with acute myocardial infarction, 23 had concurrent shock and none had died. Among them, the Yang collapse type was treated with Sin Ni Tang. It is believed that Si Ni Tang has the effect of elevating blood pressure, offering cardiotonic effects, and can resolve the problem of blood pressure drops because of a long period of time with elevated blood pressure medicine.

Shanghai Journal of Traditional Chinese Medicine (1960; 1:14): Rescued 136 serious cases of measles pneumonia, all of which were severe, complicated with infectious shock, were treated with Si Ni Tang, only 7 deaths, greatly improving the cure rate.

Tai Yin Lung Syndrome

Symptoms: General condition becomes worse, fever, restlessness, fatigue, chilly, thirsty, cough with increasing severity, wheezing with tightness or pain in the chest, profuse phlegm which may be watery, yellowish, smelly, and sometimes with blood or abscess.

Cough and wheezing with interior heat:

Ma Huang Xing Ren Gan Cao Shi Gao Tang.

Ma Huang tang (Ephedra decoction)

Ma Huang	Ephedra Sinica Stapf	6g
Xing Ren	Semen Armeniacae Amarum	12g
Shi Gao	Gypsum Fibrosum	24g
Zhi Gan Cao	Glycyrrhiza Uralensis	6g

Cough and wheezing with interior dampness:

Ma Huang Xing RenYi Ren Gan cao Tang.

Ma Huang	Ephedra Sinica Stapf	6g
Xing Ren	Semen Armeniacae Amarum	12g
Yi Yi Ren	SemenCoicis	15g
Zhi Gan Cao	Glycyrrhiza Uralensis	6g

With watery phlegm, chest distention, cough and wheezing, with edema around the eyes, and floating pulse.

Yue Bi Jia Ban Xia Tang (Yue Maidservant plus Pinellia decoction)

Ma Huang	Ephedra Sinica Stapf	6g
Sheng Jiang	Zingiber Officinale	12g
Ban Xia	Pinellia	15g
Shi Gao	Gypsum Fibrosum	20g
Da Zao	Ziziphus Jujuba Mill	9g
Zhi Gan Cao	Glycyrrhiza Uralensis	6g

With a choking cough, forceful wheezing, inability to lie down, chest distention, stress, edemoa around the eyes, limbs and whole body, runny nose, stuffy nose, loss of taste and smell add:

COVID-19 a TCM Perspective

Ting Li Da Zao Xie Fei Tang (Ting Li Da Zao Lung Purge Decoction)

| Ting Li Zi | Draba nemorosal L | 15g |
| Da Zao | Ziziphus Jujuba Mill | 9g |

With turbid stubborn phlegm, coughing, wheezing, profuse phlegm, forced to sit, not lie down and difficulty sleeping add:

Zao Jia Wan (Laundry Nut turbid phlegm moving Pill)

| Zao Jiao | Gleditsia sinensis | 9g |
| Da Zao 6 | Ziziphus Jujuba Mill | 9g |

With cough, chest tightness, turbid and bloody phlegm, abscess, fever, restlessness, chilly, thirsty, add:

Wei Jin Tang (Wei Jin Lung Abscess Decoction)

Wei Jin	Cortaderia selloana	30g
Yi Yi Ren	SemenCoicis	15g
Dong Gua Ren	Semen Benincasae	15g
Tao Ren	Semen Persicae	15g

With fluid retention (Pleural Effusion) add:

Ji Jiao Li Huang Wan (Ji Jiao Li Huang Pleural Effusion Decoction)

Fang Ji	Stephaniae Tetrandrae Radix	15g
Jiao Mu	Semen Zanthoxylum Bungeanum	12g
Ting Li Zi	Draba nemorosal L	15g
Da Huang	Rheum Palmatum	12g

Or Shi Zao Tang. (Ten Dates Decoction)

Da Ji	Euphorbia peplus Linn	15g
Yuan Hua	Genkwa Flos	12g
Gan Sui	Kansui Radix	12g
Da Zao	Ziziphus Jujuba Mill	10 pieces

With Chest Binding Syndrome结胸证:

Small Chest Binding Syndrome (小结胸证), pericarditis, myocarditis add:

Xiao Xian Xiong Tang (Minor Chest-Draining Decoction)

Huang Lian	Coptis Salisb	15g
Ban Xia	Pinellia	15g
Gua Lou Ren	Semen Trichosanthis	15g

Big Chest Binding Syndrome大结胸证, pericardial effusion add

Da Xian Xiong Wan (Major Chest-Draining Decoction)

Da Huang	Rheum Palmatum	15g
Mang Xiao	Natrii Sufas	12g
Ting Li Zi	Draba nemorosal L	15g
Xing Ren	Semen Armeniacae Amarum	12g
Gan Sui	Kansui Radix	12g
White Honey	Rectus mellis	20g

Recovery period (Pulmonary Fibrosis肺痿)

Cough with discomfort throat and chest, Fatigue.

Mai Men Dong Tang

Ban Xia	Pinellia	15g
Ren Shen	Panax ginseng C.A.Mey	12g

Gan Cao	Glycyrrhiza Uralensis	6g
Da Zao	Ziziphus Jujuba Mill	9g
Gen Mi	Oryza Sativa L	25g
Mai Meng Dong	Othiopogon japonicus	15g

Comment:

Depending on how strong the evil qi is, bronchitis and pneumonia can start at the Tai Yin stage directly. More commonly it will develop through the three Yang stages, after transforming into fire toxin. At this point the Lung is damaged and shows dysfunction with cough and/or wheezing, even Lung abscess (Lobar Pneumonia even pulmonary abscess).

You may also find that these formulas lack antibiotic qualities like herbs or other formulas to clear heat fire-toxin. It wasn't until the Yuan Dynasty, Dr. Liu Wanshu's theory that all six evil qi will eventually transform into heat-fire toxins. Later generations developed the Wen Bing School, and added formulas like Huang Lian Jie Du Tang (Huang Lian, Huang Qin, Huang bai, Zhi Zi, the earliest antibiotic-like formula) to Shang Han formulas like Ma Huang Tang. Clinical results were improving. When the first antibiotic, Penicillin (1929) and Sulfa-pyridine (1935) were created, a revolutionary change happened, but after protracted and frequent use of antibiotics, new challenges arose. As bacteria have evolved, we now see secondary infections, tolerance and diminished effectiveness with some antibiotics. Many studies show that herbal formulas have synergistic effects with antibiotics.

Ma Xing Shi Gan Tang is the most popular formula used for bronchitis and pneumonia due to bacteria and various viruses including COVID-19, therefore a lot of pharmacological research has been done.

Antitussive, relief wheezing, and anti-allergic effect.

Animal experiments have found that Ma Xing Shi Gan Tang has an anti-allergic, anti-cough and relieves wheezing. Li Jianchun found that the extract of Ma Xing Shi Gan Tang can significantly inhibit the release of histamine in the mast cells of rats, but also protects rats from antigen attack (P<0.001). The extract of Ma Xing Shi Gan Tang reduced cough by stimulating male guinea pigs with pig hair tracheal wall contact or electrical stimulation of a dog's trachea with an obvious antitussive effect. Ma Xing Shi Gan Tang works on bronchial muscle with an antihistamine effect, its effect is similar to disodium cromoglycate.

Antiviral antibacterial effect

Experiments showed that Ma Xing Shi Gan Tang has antibacterial, antiviral properties and enhances the body's immune function. Modern medical research has proved that the preparation can reduce the synthesis of bacterial proteins, destroy bacterial microstructures, and inhibit the growth of bacteria and viruses. Experiments have shown that Ma Xing Shi Gan Tang has obvious antibacterial effect on Staphylococcus aureus and Pseudomonas aeruginosa, all of which the minimum concentration of anti-Staphylococcus aureus is 1:240 and the minimum concentration of anti-green sepsis is 1:60. The main herb Ma Huang of Ma Xing Shi Gan Tang in vitro can inhibit Streptococcus A, B and other bacillus, it also has antibacterial effects. The in vitro of Ma Xing Shi Gan Tang is proven to have an inhibitory effect on the chicken embryo Shaanxi 61-1 influenza virus, and the minimum concentration of the antiviral was 1:8. 267% of Ma Xing Shi Gan Tang solution fed mice, 0. 4 mL/d for 8 days can improve the phagocytosis rate of celiac macrophils in mice (P<0.001), promoting lymphocyte conversion.

Effects on cytokines

A study on the regulation of Th1/Th2 in airway-reactive inflammatory mice by successfully establishing an asthma model in mice and observing the pulmonary alveoli irrigation and peripheral plasma IL-4 and IFN-γ concentration, found that Ma Xing Shi Gan Tang can significantly reduce the concentration of IL-4 (P<0.01) in asthma mice, and significantly improve IFN-γ, IL-12, IL-IL 18 concentration (P<0.01), after treatment, it was found that Ma Xing Shi Gan Tang can reduce the concentration of BALF and peripheral blood IL-4 in asthma mice, improve BALF and peripheral blood IFN-γ The concentration of the γ/IL-4 ratio increased significantly compared to the asthma group (P<0.01), suggesting that Ma Xing Shi Gan Tang had the effect of correcting the Th1/Th2 imbalance.

To explore the effects on targets and signal pathways of Ma Xing Shi Gan (MXSG) Decoction, and to elaborate on its possible mechanisms in the treatment of COVID-19, the active ingredients of traditional Chinese medicines of MXSG Decoction were searched from the TCMSP and TCMID database. COVID-19 targets were obtained from the GeneCards and NCBI databases. A protein-protein interaction (PPI) network was constructed through the STRING database. Cytoscape 3.7.2 software was used to create a drug-component-target-disease network. Bioconductor bioinformatics software package was used to perform gene ontology (GO) function enrichment and Kyoto encyclopedia of genes and genomes (KEGG) pathway analysis.

Results showed that MXSG Decoction contains four herbs, 127 compounds, and 237 corresponding targets. The targets of the main active ingredients of MXSG Decoction intersected with the therapeutic targets of COVID-19, obtaining 49 key targets. GO functional enrichment analysis yielded 155 GO entries (P<0.01), and KEGG pathway enrichment analysis generated 90 signal pathways (P<0.01). Construction of a drug-component-target-disease network indicated that nine compounds (e.g. quercetin, naringenin and luteolin) played a key role in the entire network.

The conclusion used the PPI network analysis and found MXSG Decoction acting on COVID-19 through key molecular targets, such as IL-6, TNF, MAPK8, MAPK3, CASP3, TP53, IL-10, CXCL8, MAPK1, CCL2, IL-1β, IL-4, PTGS2, etc. Among which, IL-6 is currently a clinical early-warning indicator for severe COVID-19 diagnosis and one of the major therapeutic targets. These targets participate cooperatively in the regulation of multiple signaling pathways, such as AGE-RAGE signaling pathway in diabetic complications, IL-17, and TNF signaling pathway, thereby exerting anti-inflammatory, antiviral and immune-regulatory effects. (Network pharmacological study on mechanism of Maxing Shigan Decoction in treatment of coronavirus disease 2019 (COVID-19),[J]. Chinese Herbal Medicine. 2020, 51(8):1996-2003

Ting Li Da Zao Lung Purge Decoction is the most common formula for Heart function failure when there is pneumonia. In order to explore the mechanism, based on network pharmacology, high-resolution mass spectrometry and molecular docking technology, the active ingredients and mechanisms of the treatment of Heart failure by Ting Li Da Zao Xie Fei Tang were discussed. Methods: Through literature review and combined with the BATMAN-TCM database, the two herbs of Chinese medicine ingredients and drug targets in Ting Li Da Zao Xie Fei Tang were retrieved. Using Heart failure as the key word, the GeneCards database is used to collect targets for Heart failure disease, the common target based on drug and disease uses STORING data platform to analyze protein-protein interaction (PPI), and network complement analysis through Cytoscape software, and finally obtains the core target. Based on the core target, the Kyoto Gene and Genomic encyclopedia (KEGG) pathway enrichment analysis is carried out through the DAVID database, and a drug-component-target-path molecular network is established. Based on the results of the above network pharmacology research, the high-resolution mass spectrometry technology was used to analyze the decoction and confirm the selected active ingredients. The autoDock 4.2.6 software is used to verify molecular docking of key active ingredients and related targets.

Results: A total of 85 components of Ting Li Zi were obtained, 49 components of Da Zao, 1,078 drug targets, 1,549 disease targets and 262 common targets. After protein interaction analysis and network complement analysis, 23 core targets and 33 active ingredients were obtained, involving 19 signaling pathways (P<0.05). The results of mass spectrometry show that 18 components, molecular docking analysis results indicate that six core components and silent information regulation factor 1 (SIRT1), albumocyte mediate (IL) 1B, protein kinase B alpha (AKT1), tumor necrosis factor (TNF) have better binding activity; The process of compound overall intervention to treat Heart failure mainly involves signaling pathways such as MAPK, hypoxic induction factor-1 (HIF-1), and rapamycin target protein (mTOR).

Conclusion: The study initially revealed the active ingredients and mechanism of anti-Heart failure effects in Ting Li Da Zao Xie Fei Tang, it provided reference for guiding the screening of quality control markers of Ting Li Da Zao Xie Fei Tang, and the discovery of the active ingredients. Zhao Jie etc. Analysis of the active ingredients and mechanisms of the anti-Heart failure effect in Ting Li Da Zao Xie Fei Tang based on network pharmacology and mass spectrometry analysis. [J]Chinese Journal of Experimental Prescription Pharmacy. Chinese Academy of Traditional Chinese Medicine, Zunyi Medical University.Volume 27, 2021, No. 8, pp. 151-160

Ji Jiao Li Huang Wan is an expanded version of Ting Li Da Zao Xie Fei Tang used for treatment and prevention of pneumonia complicated with pleural effusion, Heart functional failure and Lung functional failure, in Ji Jiao Li Huang Wan, Ting Li Zi can lower pulmonary blood pressure with a cardiotonic effect, and a diuretic effect. Fang Ji and Jiao Mu enhance the diuretic effect and can lower the Heart's extra burden. It can treat or prevent Heart function failure. Da Huang purges the bowels can lower abdominal cavity pressure, improve diaphragm movement, and improve respiratory function to prevent Lung functional failure.

5. Shaoyin syndrome and Treatment

Symptoms and Signs: Being sleepy suddenly after irritability, poor reaction time, unclear mind, listlessness before unconsciousness, feeble, thread-like, disappearing pulse.

1. Shao Yin syndrome with cold-deficiency type: suddenly complaining of aversion to cold, curling up to keep warm, extremely cold limbs with cold sweating, unclear mind, listlessness before becoming unconscious, strong desire to sleep, feeble and thready pulse, may have watery diarrhea with undigested food, cold urine.

Si Ni Tang (Frigid Extremities Decoction)

Warm up Heart and Kidney Yang, rescue collapse

Fu Zi	Aconiti Lateralis Radix Praeparata	15g
Gan Jiang	Zingiber Officinale	12g
Zhi Gan Cao	Glycyrrhiza Uralensis	6g

(2) Shao Yin syndrome with deficiency-heat type: Irritability, sleeplessness, dry mouth and throat, red tongue, scanty fur, and thread rapid pulse.

Huang Lian E Jiao Tang (Coptis Donkey Skin Glue Decoction)

Huang Lian	Coptis Salisb	15g
Huang Qin	Scutellaria baicalensis Georgi	12g
Bai Shao Yao	Paeonia Lactiflora	12g
E Jiao	Asini Corii Colla	15g
Chicken Egg		2 pieces

(3) Shao Yin syndrome with edema: Edema all over the body, difficult urination, palpitations, dizziness, shivering all over the body, tendency to fall down, heaviness sensation and pain in the limbs, may have diarrhea and lower abdominal pain.

Zhen Wu Tang (Hero Zhen Wu Decoction for Edema)

Fu Zi	Aconiti Lateralis Radix Praeparata	15g
Gan Jiang	Zingiber Officinale	12g
Bai Zhu	Atractylodes Macrocephala	12g
Fu Ling	Poria	12g
Bai Shao Yao	Paeonia Lactiflora	12g

Comment

When the disease reaches the Shao Yin stage (Related to Heart and Kidney), the situation is most likely critical. Some of the symptomology in this pattern can seem unusual at first glance. Listed as suddenly becoming tired after being irritable, having poor reactions and an unclear mind refers to a progressive set of symptoms experienced by the patient as well as the people around them. The irritability and sleepiness happen on the patient's side, while the poor reaction refers to how caregivers or family members may react to the patient's behavior. Finally, the patient's mind becomes unclear in response to being quite ill at this advanced stage. The further progression includes listlessness, drop in blood pressure etc. All of these indicate an emergency condition like Heart failure or toxic shock due to Heart and Kidney Yang collapse. At this point the patient is actively dying. Si Ni Tang which contains cardiotonic alkaloid aconitine is assumed to be the first cardiotonic agent in medical science history and is a very effective rescuer. It is still popularly used in the emergency department in TCM hospitals in China as an injection.

If the patient survives this stage, then it may become a chronic condition due to Kidney Yin damage and deficient heat. There may be anxiety, or chronic insomnia. Kidney Yang may also be damaged as a result. There may be edema due to chronic nephritis or chronic nephritic syndrome. Huang Lian E jiaoTang is a very effective formula for treating psychological disorders post-infection, and Zhen Wu Tang, named by hero Zhen Wu who defeated flood at remote ancient time, is always a good formula for edema due to Kidney damage from plagues.

To summarize, the progress of applied research on the treatment of Kidney disease with Zhen Wu Tang, Liu Qiri et al. collected and summarized the articles on the treatment of Kidney disease and the intervention of animal experiments of Kidney disease with Zhen Wu Tang in the past 10 years. Results were Zhen Wu Tang is a classic warm yang formula to eliminate water, which can be used in cardiovascular diseases, digestive diseases, urinary diseases and so on. In relation to Kidney disease, Zhen Wu Tang can be used to treat chronic nephritis, chronic renal failure, nephritic syndrome, diabetic Kidney disease, Heart and Kidney syndrome, etc.

Gao Min used Zhen Wu Tang to treat 120 cases of Spleen and Kidney yang deficiency type chronic glomerulonephritis based on controlling infection, lowering blood pressure, protecting Kidney function and correcting the balance of hydro-electrolyte acid and alkali. The clinical efficacy of the Zhen Wu Tang group was as high as 93.3%, and the total relief rate was 60.0%.

Creatinine, urea nitrogen, and urinary protein were reduced compared to those who did not take Zhen Wu Tang. Sun Xixuan used Zhen Wu Tang to treat diabetic Kidney disease in a controlled trial of 130 cases, the results show that the treatment group after treatment using Chinese medicine improved more obviously, the effective rate of the treatment group was 90.77 percent, higher than the control group. After treatment, creatinine removal rate, urine protein quantification, fasting blood sugar and serum creatinine decreased significantly, with more advantages than the control group. Zeng Wei Ping test results show that Zhen Wu Tang can reduce the rate of urine albumin excretion, reduce the expression of endothelial cell growth factors in blood vessels, and have the function of protecting the Kidneys. The results of the treatment of chronic renal failure in stage III-IV with Zhen Wu Tang showed that the effectiveness of the treatment group reached 79.31 percent, which was significantly improved compared with the control group, and the 24h urine protein quantification, Scr.urea nitrogen was reduced, and the levels of CTGF and HGF in serum were lowered. Han Ling and other research results show that Zhen Wu Tang may be by reducing the Kidney damage-related factors to reduce the role of renal interstitial fibrosis. In the experiment, the urine KIM-1, clusterin and OPN of the rats in the experimental group were significantly reduced. Liu Meifang used mate analysis of 10 treatments of primary nephrotic syndrome randomized controlled trials. The results show that the effect of Zhen Wu Tang treatment of the disease is obvious, it can reduce 24h urine protein quantification, increase serum albumin, reduce total serum cholesterol, serum triglycerides, hematopolycerin.

Conclusion: The treatment of Kidney disease in Zhen Wu Tang has a remarkable effect, which can improve the clinical symptoms of patients, and has the effect of reducing toxin accumulation in the body, improving blood circulation, improving the pathological state of the Kidneys and protecting Kidney function. *Advances in the treatment of Kidney disease with Zhen Wu Tang*, Liu Ruiqi, Chen Bozhi. Tianjin University of Traditional Chinese Medicine. Nei Mongol Journal of Traditional Chinese Medicine. 2019(06) Page:158-160

6.Jueyin syndrome and Treatment

Symptoms and Signs: excessive thirst, rebellious qi (Nausea, Vomiting), pain and heat in the Heart and Stomach, hunger but with no desire to eat, possible vomiting of roundworm after forced eating, and continual diarrhea.

(1) Simultaneous occurrence of cold and heat syndrome, with symptoms of vexation, May experience vomiting after eating, even vomiting roundworm, cold limbs, abdominal pain, cold sweat.

Wu Mei Pill (Dark Plum Fruit Pill)

Wu Mei	Mume Fructus	15g
Chuan Jiao	Zanthoxylum Bungeanum Maxim	12g
Fu Zi	Aconiti Lateralis Radix Praeparata	15g
Gan Jiang	Zingiber Officinale	12g
Zhi Gan Cao	Glycyrrhiza Uralensis	6g
Xi Xin	Asarum Sieboldii Miq	9g
Huang Lian	Coptis Salisb	15g
Huang Bai	Cortex Phellodendri Chinensis	15g
Ren Shen	Panax ginseng C.A.Mey	12g
Dang Gui	Angelica Sinensis	12g

(2). High fever, unconsciousness, convulsion, diarrhea, yellowish, smelly, sticky stool with blood, abscess, mucosa, abdominal pain, rectal tenesmus, hot sensation around anus, thirsty.

Bai Tou Weng Tang (White Hair Grandpa Dysentery Decoction)

Bai Tou Weng	Radix Pulsatillae	20g
Huang Bai	Cortex Phellodendri Chinensis	15g
Huang Lian	Coptis Salisb	15g
Qin Pi	Franxini Cortex	15g

Comment

In the Jue Yin stage, Dr. Zhang Zhongjing listed this disease as severe acute gastroenteritis causing burning abdominal pain, diarrhea, vomiting, dehydration. Protracted inflammation can lead to poor circulation leading to Yang deficiency symptoms like cold limbs, excessive thirst that may get better after drinking water, cold sweats, convulsion, unclear consciousness even unconsciousness due to invasion of Pericardium and Liver. This pattern is referred to as a simultaneous occurrence of cold and heat syndrome. This is the original indication for Wu Mei Wan, even though this formula has been used in clinic often for painful shock due to roundworm invading the biliary ducts causing so-called roundworm fainting (Hui Jue 蛔厥) as well.

When Shang Han transforms into a fire-heat toxin, it reaches the Jue Yin Stage, it will manifest as a higher fever, chilly, unconsciousness, convulsion, stiff and rolled tongue, contracted scrotum etc., brain damage. Toxic bacillary dysentery is a good example, which can start with unconsciousness and convulsions, even before diarrhea with bloody abscess. Bai Tou Weng Tang is supposed to be the first effective antibiotic-like anti-dysentery formula in medical science history. It had been selected and listed in the Jue Yin chapter by Dr. Zhang Zhongjing.

Research has shown that Bai Tou weng Tang has a strong antibacterial effect, no matter in vitro or in vivo. Furthermore, it has anti-amoeba protozoa, and anti-inflammatory effects, it enhances immune function and other effects.

1. Antibacterial: Bai Tou Weng Tang has an obvious inhibitory effect on Shiga and other dysentery bacteria. For staphylococcus aureus, epidermal staphylococcus and cartacoccus it also has a strong antibacterial effect. It also has an obvious inhibition effect on skin fungi. Among Bai Tou Weng Tang on dysentery bacteria inhibition, Huang Lian, Qin Pi is the strongest, Huang Bai is second, Bai Tou Weng is the weakest.

2. Anti-amoeba protozoa: Bai Tou Weng Tang has an anti-amoeba protozoa effect, decoction and its saponin effect is more obvious, high concentration can completely inhibit its growth.

3. Anti-inflammatory: Bai Tou Weng Tang was used in a variety of experiments on rats' claw puffiness and granuloma. Local use can reduce the development of granuloma, the effect is like butazolidin.

4. Enhanced immune function: Bai Tou Weng Tang can enhance the ability of white blood cells cytophagy on Staphylococcus aureus and can enhance the phagocytosis function of the endothelial system. For bacterial toxins, it also has a significant detoxification effect, which can undoubtedly promote the body's function and enhance disease resistance.

Enema with Bai Tou Weng Tang for 34 cases of dysentery patients started to work in 1-5 days. Symptoms of abdominal pain and tenesmus disappeared in about 1 day on average, diarrhea took 3 days. 30 cases were cured, 4 cases were improved, the efficiency rate was 100%. Retained enemas with Bai Tou Weng Tang treated 136 cases of amoeba bowel disease. Results: Cured (clinical symptoms disappeared, stool culture 3 consecutive times, amoeba culture are negative, follow-up 1 year did not relapse) 128 cases, effective (clinical symptoms basically disappeared, stool culture amoeba trophozoite negative, after discontinuation of medicine there are still abdominal pain, urinal) 6 cases, No effect 2 cases. Total efficiency is 98%.

In a study of the treatment of cases of salmonella enteritis with Bai Tou Weng Tang, of the 76 patients, 62 cases of fever disappeared time was 0.5-6 days, dehydration corrected time was an average of 3.2 days, diarrhea or pus disappeared was 2.5-9 days, an average of 4.2 days; There were 75 cases of discharge from hospital and 1 case died of multiple organ failure from sepsis.

Bai Tou Weng Tang is a very effective antibiotic-like formula for dysentery, it has been a traditional and classic formula for toxic dysentery since Shang Han Lun nearly 2000 year ago. Regarding heat fire toxin entering the Jueyin Pericardium causing unconsciousness and convulsions due to brain damage and entering Jueyin Liver result in heat fire toxin in Ying level and blood level as disseminated intravenous coagulation (DIC), which often lead to multiple inner organs functional failure. After that, the other TCM doctors had well developed Warmth Plague theory (Wen Bing Theory) and better formulas to deal with, which formed Wen Bing School.

Wen Bing School:

Wei Qi Ying Xue Syndrome Differentiation and Treatment System

Three Jiao Syndrome Differentiation and Treatment System

The Shang Han school focused on cold induced plagues. There was more emphasis on the three Yang stages. Detail was lacking especially in reference to the Jue Yin stage. At the end of the Ming Dynasty and beginning of the Qing Dynasty a growing, concentrated population and urbanization process was well under way. In particular, the northern nomads and the southern farming civilizations migrated, creating the north-south integration. More people lived in Southern China in large cities along the Yangtze River where the weather is hot and humid. China's population was 150 million at the end of the Ming Dynasty, and finally reached 400 million by 1833AD,. Increased frequent commercial exchanges, plus warm climate, allowed more warm-induced plagues to appear. Ones such as Epidemic Meningitis, Encephalitis, Epidemic Hemorrhagic Fever, Measles, Chickenpox, Scarlet fever, smallpox etc. This created the need for the Wei, Qi Ying, Xue syndrome differentiation and treatment system as well as the Three Jiao differentiation and treatment system. The core theories of the Wen Bing School are discussed below.

Wei Qi Ying Xue Syndrome differentiation and Treatment

There are different kinds of Wen Bing, named respectively: Wind Warmth, Spring Warmth, Summer heat warmth, Dampness Warmth, Autumn Dryness warmth, Hidden summer warmth, Winter Warmth, and Warm toxin.

Wei Qi Ying Xue describes the four common stages of the Wen Bing mentioned above. These all have different locations, different severity, and different prognosis.

1. Wei level syndrome and Treatment

Wen Bing warmth evil first attacks the wei level, leading to Lung and defensive system dysfunction.

Symptoms and signs: Fever, no aversion to cold, sweating, sore throat, thirst, cough, red tongue, white thin coat, floating, rapid pulse.

Principle of treatment: Release exterior with acrid cool, clear heat and toxine.

Yin Qiao San (Golden-and-silver Honeysuckle & Forsythia powder)

Jin Yin Hua	Lonicera Japonica Thunb	15g
Lian Qiao	Forsythia suspensa	15g
Niu Bang zi	Arctii Fructus	12g
Bo He	Menta piperita	12g
Jing Jie Hui	Schizonepetae Spica	9g
Dan Dou Shi	Sojae Semen Praeparatum	9g
Dan zhu Ye	Lophatherum gracile	12g
Jie Geng	Platycodon grandiflorus	12g
Lu Gen	Phragmitis Rhizoma	20g
Gan Cao	Glycyrrhiza Uralensis	6g

Comment

Like Ma Huang Tang for cold induced plagues in Shang Han Lun, Yin Qiao San is the most representative formula for initial stage warmth induced plagues in the Wen Bing School. Unlike Ma Huang Tang, Yin Qiao San is led by the king herb Jin Yin Hua and Lian Qiao which are acrid and cool in nature, not only can they release exterior wind-heat, it can also clear heat and toxins.

Modern pharmaceutical research have shown that the active ingredients chlorogenic acid and caffeic acid found in honeysuckle can bind with neuraminidase and surround influenza viruses, thereby inhibiting replication of viruses at an early stage [7]. Another newly discovered active ingredient miRNA-miR2911 can inhibit H1N1, H5N1 and H7N9 in vitro and in vivo especially in the Lungs [8]. There are inhibitory effects on adenoviruses, Herpes virus, Echo, Coxsackie virus etc, also on bacteria-like staphylococcus aureus, pneumococcus, streptococcus, E-coli, Bacillus dysenteriae, Bacillus typhi, paratyphoid bacilli, Bacillus pertussis, Diplococcus meningitidis etc.

Forsythia phenol has a synergistic effect with honeysuckle on various influenza viruses like rhinovirus etc, bacteria as well, including staphylococcus aureus, pneumococcus, streptococcus, Bacillus diphtheriae, Bacillus pestis, Tubercle bacillus, Leptospira etc. For H7N9, the Forsythia group was better than the control group with Oseltamivir.[9].

Recent studies indicate that the active ingredient from Gan Cao can inhibit replication of corona viruses (IC50=0.27mg/ml) [10], and bind with ACE2, raw Gan Cao is traditionally used for clearing heat and fire toxins.

Yin Qiao San has been utilized for a long time in China for epidemic diseases at the early stage like common cold, variations of Flu A, B, H1N1, H7N9 etc., and scarlet fever. More recently, for SARS, COVD-19, it remains one of the most popular and effective formulas in the clinic and at home in the personal medicine cabinet.

2. Qi level syndrome and Treatment

Evil from Wei Level transforms and becomes interior heat, interior heat blazing. The battle between evil and vital qi is severe at this level. The Qi level syndrome includes the following.

(1). Heat in the Qi Level:

High fever, red face, profuse sweating, irritability, strong thirst, red tongue and flooding pulse. This pattern is like Yang Ming Syndrome in the Shang Han Lun.

Clear Qi level heat, drain Stomach fire, generate body fluid and alleviate thirst.

Bai Hu Tang. (White Tiger Decoction)

Shi Gao	Gypsum Fibrosum	24g
Zhi Mu	Anemarrhenae Rhizoma	15g
Stick rice	Oryza Sativa L	25g
Gan Cao	Glycyrrhiza Uralensis	6g

(2). Heat and fire blocking the Lung

Fever, cough, wheezing, chest discomfort or pain, yellowish phlegm, red tongue, yellow even grey black coating. Rapid and slippery pulse.

Clear Lung heat fire, resolve phlegm, descent Lung Qi.

Ma Xing Shi Gan Tang

Ma Huang tang (Ephedra decoction)

Ma Huang	Ephedra Sinica Stapf	6g
Xing Ren	Semen Armeniacae Amarum	12g
Shi Gao	Gypsum Fibrosum	24g
Zhi Gan Cao	Glycyrrhiza Uralensis	6g

Add: Jin Yin hua, Liao Qiao, Yu Xin Cao, Huang Qin, Gua Lou, Zhe Bei Mu

(3). Heat blocking the Stomach and intestines

Lung heat may descend to the Stomach and intestines, resulting in high fever, aversion to heat, heavy breath, red face, and eyes, sweating, constipation with abdominal bloating, pain, agitation, delirium, red tongue with yellowish dry coating, deep and forceful pulse.

Purge heat accumulation in Yang Ming.

Da Cheng Qi Tang. (Major Order the Qi decoction)

Da Huang	Rheum Palmatum	15g
Mang Xiao	Natrii Sulfas	12g
Zhi Shi	Citrus aurantium	12g
Huo Po	Magnolia Officinalis	12g

Comment

The fight between vital qi and evil qi is worse at the Qi level. It is most likely complicated with a bacterial infection, resulting in complications like pharyngitis, laryngitis, Sinusitis, Otitis Media etc. Endotoxin from bacteria leads to a condition of deterioration manifesting as the four big symptoms synonymous with Yang Ming Syndrome: high fever, sweating, thirsty, and flood pulse.

Clinically, epidemic diseases, especially respiratory epidemics like Flu, Measles, Chicken pox, SARS, MERS, even COVID-19 always attack initially in the upper respiratory tract (Tai Yang stage in Shang Han or Wei stage in Wen Bing). Then they get into the lower respiratory tract and acute bronchitis, even pneumonia (Tai Yin Lung or Qi level in Wen Bing since there are still four big symptoms and signs). Cough and wheezing become prevalent due to Lung dysfunction. When heat-fire toxins worsen, they will move to the Stomach and intestines leading to higher fever, delirium, constipation, severe abdominal distention and pain, a toxic paralytic intestinal obstruction happens.

As an antibiotic-like, strong antipyretic, anti-inflammatory formula, White Tiger Decoction Bai Hu Tang is best for Wen Bing heat at the Qi level. If bronchitis or pneumonia occurs, Ma Xing Shi Gan Tang is the first choice, even for SARS, COVID-19.

A total of 2 articles on Covid-19 described trials using Lotus flower Clear Heat Capsule. (Lian Hua Qing Wen Capsule is a patent formula modified from Ma Xing Shi Gan Tang with Honeysuckle & Forsythia). The studies included 154 patients. All the participating patients were diagnosed with new coronavirus pneumonia (COVID-19). The meta-analysis results showed that the disappearance rate of the main clinical symptoms using Chinese medicine Lianhua Qingwen in the treatment of new coronavirus pneumonia was significantly higher than that of the control group [OR = 3.34, 95% CI (2.06, 5.44), P <0.001]; the disappearance rate of other clinical secondary symptoms is significantly higher than the control group [OR = 6.54, 95% CI (3.59, 11.90), P <0.001]. The duration of fever was significantly lower than that of the control group [OR = -1.04, 95% CI (-1.60, -0.49), P <0.001]. It is confirmed that the traditional Chinese medicine Lianhua Qingwen treatment improves clinical effectiveness and has certain advantages in relieving cough and fever. [11]

When toxic paralytic intestinal obstruction is present, which Dr.Zhang Zhongjing called Yang Ming Organ syndrome in the Shang Han Lun, the best formula is still the Shang Han purgative formula Da Chen Qi Tang.

As you can see, the Wen Bing School had inherited a lot of academic thought and formulas from the Shang Han School. The real revolutionary development of the Wen Bing School is its discussion of the JueYin Pericardium and Liver stage (Yin and Blood level in Wen Bing School). The patient starts to present unconsciousness due to brain damage, and heat toxin in Liver yin and blood which cause DIC resulting in death due to multiple inner organ failure. For some reason, maybe the Shang Han Lun was lost, we cannot find this part in the remaining Shang Han Lun, and it was the Wen Bing School who developed this information.

Ying level syndrome and Treatment. For severe cases, Qi level interior heat may become heat-fire toxin, and enter into the Ying level, located in the Pericardium and Liver. When body fluids are damaged, blood is more viscous and stagnated. Interior heat fire toxin forces blood out of the blood vessels, manifesting as bleeding under the skin and looks like macula, this is the beginning of Disseminated Intravenous Coagulation (DIC). Pericardium dysfunction shows more cognitive and mental problems stemming from brain damage.

Heat at the Ying Level (beginning of DIC)

General condition has deteriorated, fever becomes worse at night, irritability, increasing delirium, delusion, even unconsciousness, bleeding like a macula under skin, deep red crimson tongue, thin and rapid pulse.

Clean heat, cool ying, reverse from ying level to qi level.

Qing Ying Tang (Clear the Nutritive Level Decoction)

Xi Jiao	Rhinoceros sondaicus	12g
Shen Di Huang	Radix Rehmanniae	15g
Dan Shen	Salvia miltiorrhiza	15g
Jin Yin Hua	Lonicera Japonica	15g
Liao Qiao	Forsythia suspensa	15g
Huang Lian	Coptis Salisb	12g
Dan Zhu Ye	Lophatherum gracile	12g
Xuan sheng	Scrophularia ningpoensis	12g
Mai Meng Dong	Othiopogon japonicus	15g

Studies have shown that Qing Ying Tang has an anti-inflammatory, anti-infective effect. One study used animal intravenous endotoxin to cause heat in the ying blood model to research Qing Ying Tang's effect. The results showed that it can significantly inhibit endotoxin causing rabbit inflammatory mediator PGE2 to release 5-HT, improving serum IgG in the body, reducing the blood viscosity. It can promote the excretion of endotoxins in the body, inhibit the increase of capillaries permeability and significantly inhibit the non-specific inflammatory response of rats.

Qing Ying Tang has many pharmacological effects, including regulating body temperature, reducing blood viscosity and platelet aggregation capacity, regulating clotting and fibrosis, improving the body's antioxidant resistance, resisting the damage of free radicals, and maintaining the stability of electrolytes in the body

Qing ying tang has an obvious antipyretic effect on E. coli endotoxin in the rabbit model, it has a strong effect on improving the symptoms and lowering the body temperature of rabbits. There was research that this formula can prevent the disseminated intravascular coagulation (DIC) caused by E. coli endotoxin (Liu Xinxuan, et al. [J] Chinese Medicine and Clinical. 1995(2).

Qing Ying Tang is suitable for patients experiencing Flu, type B encephalitis, epidemic meningococcal meningitis, toxemia, sepsis etc. with early stage of DIC.

Heat entering into the Pericardium (Central Nervous System damage)

High fever, unclear mind, unconsciousness, cold extremities, seizure, deep red tongue, rapid and slippery pulse, mental disturbance, all due to heat in the Pericardium.

Formulas: An Gong Niu Huang wan (Peace palace cow bezoar pill)

   Or Zhi Bao Dan (Top treasure pill)
   Or Zi Xue Dan (Blue snow powder)

An Gong Niu HuangWan <Detailed analysis on febrile diseases>温病条辨

(Peace palace cow bezoar pill)

Niu Huang	Bos Taurus domesticus	12g
Shui Niu Jiao	Cornu Bubali	24g
She Xiang	Moschus	2g
Zhen Zhu	Margarita	9g
Zhu Sha	Cinnabaris	6g
Xiong Huang	Crocosmia Planch	6g
Huang Lian	Coptis Salisb	15g
Huang Qin	Scutellaria baicalensis Georgi	12g
Zhi Zi	Gardenia Elli, nom, cons	15g
Yu Jin	Curcumae Radix	12g
Bing Pian	Borneolum Syntheticum	9g

Zhi Bao Dan

(Top treasure pill)

Xi Jiao	Cornu Rhinoceri	12g
Dai Mao	Carapax Eretmochelydis	12g
Hu Bo	Succinum	9g
Zhu Sha	Cinnabaris	6g
Xiong Huang	Crocosmia Planch	6g
Niu Huang	Bos Taurus domesticus	12g
Long Nao	Borneolum Syntheticum	9g
She Xiang	Moschus	2g
An Xi Xiang	Styrax benzoin	9g
Golden Paper	Native gold	0.2g
Silver Paper	Native silver	0.2g

Zi Xue Dan (Blue snow powder)

Shi Gao	Gypsum Fibrosum	30g
Hua Shi	Talcum	20g
Han Shui Shi	Gypsum Rubrum	20g
Ci Shi	Magnetium Magnetite	3g
Niu Jiao	Cornu Bubali	24g
Ling Yang Jiao	Saiga tatarica Linnaeus	12g
Chen Xiang	Aquilariasinensis (Lour.) spreng	9g
Qing Mu Xiang	Radix Aristolochiae	12g
Xuan Sheng	Scrophularia ningpoensis Hemsl	12g
Shen Ma	Rhizoma Cimicifugae	12g
Zhi Gan cao	Glycyrrhiza Uralensis	6g
Ding Xiang	Syzygium aromaticum	12g
Mang Xiao	Natrii Sulfas	12g
She Xiang	Moschus	2g

Su He Xiang Wan

Su He Xiang	Styrax	12g
She Xiang	Moschus	6g
Bing Pian	Borneolum	9g
Mu Xiang	RX. Aucklandiae	9g
An Xi Xiang	Benzoinum	9g
Tan Xiang	Lignum Santali Albi	12g
Ru Xiang	Olibanum	9g
Ding Xiang	Flos Caryophylli	9g
Xiang Fu	Rz.Cyperi	12g
Bi Ba	Fr.Piperis Longi	6g
Xi Jiao	Cornu Rhinoceri	6g
Zhu Sha	Cinnabaris	6g
Bai Zhu	Rz.Atractylodis Macrocephalae	12g
He Zi	Fr.Chebulae	12g

Some medicinals that are derived from animals are no longer used due to laws protecting animals, some are not used due to labor protection, and some have severe toxic side effects. These include Xi Jiao, Ling Yang Jiao, Zhu Sha, Xiong Huang et. For the safety, Practitioners are advised to use patent production, where proper substitutions are used, or avoid these ingredients altogether.

Formulas used for clearing away heat and toxins, relieving convulsion and assisting resuscitation, were also used to treat heat evil invasion with high fever, restlessness, delirium, loss of consciousness with turbid phlegm and infantile febrile convulsions due to brain damage. Those treasured formulas are essentially the herbs with actions like antibiotics, anti-viral, anti-inflammatory, anti-toxin, anti-DIC.

Modern pharmacological experiments show that An Gong Niu Huang Pills has a better protective effect on acute cerebral hemorrhage and cerebral ischemic injury in rats, and it has certain positive effects on cerebral edema, cerebral ischemic hypoxia status, etc. In closed brain injury rats, it also has a certain interventional effect on rats with sepsis. Zhi Bao Dan, Zi Xue Dan have similar pharmacological functions.

Extreme Liver heat causing wind

High fever, agitate, convulsion, seizure of limbs, stiff neck, opisthotonus, shaking of tongue, may

with unconsciousness, red tongue, rapid and wiry pulse.

Treatment principle: Clean Liver heat, cool blood, calm wind

Ling Yang Gou Teng Tang (Antelope Horn & Gambir Calm Wind Decoction)

Ling Yang Jiao	Saigae Tataricae Cornu	12g
Gou Teng	Gambir Plant	9g
Sang Ye	Morus alba L	15g
Chuan Bei Mu	Fritillaria thunbergii	15g
Zhu Ru	Bambusae Caulis in Taenias	12g
Sheng Di Huang	Radix rehmanniae Recens	15g
Ju Hua	Flos Chrysanthemi	12g
Bai Shao	Paeonia Lactiflora	12g
Fu Shen	Poria cum Radix	12g
Gan Cao	Glycyrrhiza Uralensis	6g

Ling Yang Gou Teng is applied in cases when convulsions become predominant due to brain damage. It contains herbs that clear heat toxins and infection and are combined with antipyretic and convulsion relieving herbs like Ling Yang Jiao and Gou Teng.

Blood level syndrome and Treatment

This stage presents when heat in the Ying level becomes worse. This is the most critical stage and is typical in cases of DIC. Most likely there will be multiple organ failure and eventually Yang collapses and the patient will die.

Symptoms and signs: febrile disease continues to get worse, hematemesis, hematochezia, haemoptysis, hematuria, bleeding under the skin, fever especially at night, irritability, unclear mind even unconsciousness, may have convulsions, dark or purplish tongue, thin and rapid pulse.

Xi Jiao Di Huang Tang (Rhinoceros horn & rehmannia root cooling blood decoction)

Shui Niu Jiao	Buffalo horns	12g
Shen Di Huang	Radix rehmanniae Recens	15g
Chi Shao Yao	Paeonia veitchii Lynch	15g
Mu Dan Pi	Moutan Cortex	15g

Comments

Most Wen Bing diseases show the same process of development. They begin at the Wei level or Qi level. They initially attack the Lungs, then may adversely invade Jue Yin Pericardium and Liver, causing brain damage with unconsciousness, and convulsion due to Liver wind, and DIC. When heat and fire toxins reach the Ying and Blood level, it will result in bleeding, shock and multiple inner organs failure (Obstruction syndrome, Collapse syndrome in TCM). Rubella, measles, chickenpox, scarlet fever, SARS, MERS, even COVID-19 etc. all follow this law.

The Shang Han Lun is more detailed on the three Yang stages, and the Wen Bing School in the Qing Dynasty had a great breakthrough on the three Yin stages of diagnosis and treatment. Master Ye Tianshi said "generally, the opinion is that after the Wei level is Qi level, and after Ying level is the Blood level. In the initial stages release the exterior with diaphoresis, then clear heat at the Qi level. When the disease invades the blood level, one should be cautious about blood consumed and bleeding, and must only focus on cooling the blood and moving blood stasis.

Ying level disease is the beginning of DIC. It is a key point to lower severe case rate and mortality, Qing Ying Tang uses Xi Jiao, Sheng Di huang, Dan Sheng, Xuan Sheng to cool yin and blood, those can improve capillary blood circulation, counter thrombosis, while still using Jin Yin

Hua, Lian Qiao, Huang Lian to clear toxin from viruses and bacteria. Sheng Di Huang, Mai Men Dong, Xuan Sheng are used to supplement body fluids and to prevent dehydration, since toxins and dehydration can both trigger DIC and/or make it worse.

When the disease reaches the Blood level marked by various kinds of bleeding, the patient may die shortly from DIC. The DIC rescue formula Xi Jiao Di Huang Tang is a small simple formula focused on cooling the blood with Xi Jiao, Sheng Di Huang, Chi Shao Yao, Mu Dan Pi, and is a very needed effective formula.

Xi Jiao has a cardiotonic effect, it can decrease permeability of the capillary blood vessels, lowering blood pressure after first elevating blood pressure, this is normal; Sheng Di Huang can strengthen the Heart, promote urination, lower blood pressure, dilate blood vessels inside the Kidney to relieve Kidney damage, while stimulating bone marrow to elevate platelets. It can be beneficial when DIC happens; Shao Yao can antagonize ischemia in the myocardial tissue, dilate peripheral blood vessels, and inhibit platelet aggregation to reduce thrombosis; Mu Dan Pi can strongly inhibit platelet aggregation, reduce TAX2, prevent thrombosis. All of these can be beneficial in the treatment of DIC.

Xue Bi Jing injection has been permitted for use by the Chinese government COVID-19 protocol 2019-2020. A randomized, controlled trial of 710 cases results indicate that it can reduce 28 hospitalization days, significantly improving the pneumonia severity index, it can shorten mechanical ventilation time by 5.5days, ICU length of stay by 4 days. Speculation on how such good results were achieved is that it relates to improving capillary blood circulation, countering thrombosis function and preventing the cytokine storm. [12].

When there is unconsciousness due to JueYin Pericardium dysfunction causing brain damage, then the famous Wen Bing Three Treasure formulas An Gong Niu Huang wan (Peace palace cow bezoar pill), Zhi Bao Dan (Top treasure pill), Zi Xue Dan (Blue snow powder) are needed. The foundation of these formulas is to clear heat-fire toxins and cool the blood.

To these formulae add Niu Huang, She Xiang, Pin Pian to stimulate the central nervous system, open the orifice, and revive the mind.

Ling Yang Gou Teng Tang (Antelope Horn & Gambir Calm Wind Decoction) is especially designed for relieving convulsions, with the three treasures all for Jue Yin brain damage.

Three Jiao Syndrome differentiation and Treatment system

Wei Qi Ying Xue theory focuses on warmth plagues. The Three Jiao theory focuses on damp-heat Wen Bing, which starts in the Upper Jiao (Lung and Pericardium). Dr.Ye Tianshi said "Warm evil always attacks the Lung in the upper part of the body, and may adversely transfer to the Pericardium. Then it will move to the Middle Jiao (Spleen and Stomach), and finally to the Lower Jiao (Liver and Kidney). From the upper to the lower just like water moves during water metabolism. Three Jiao theory deals more with damp evil. The treatment method is to disperse in the Upper Jiao, resolve turbid with aromatics in the Middle Jiao, and eliminate dampness with tasteless diuretics. in the Lower Jiao.

Upper Jiao Syndrome differentiation and Treatment

Symptoms and signs; No aversion to cold, fever, heavy sensation on head as if wrapped in a towel, tired limbs, heaviness in the body, chest and abdominal distention and sometimes painful, vomit, nausea, diarrhea, cough, sore throat, thirst with no desire to drink. Tongue coating white or yellowish, thick and greasy. Floating and slippery pulse.

1. Cold predominate Pattern:

Huo Xiang Zheng Qi San (Agastache Anti-Stomach Flu Powder)

Huo Xiang	Agastache rugosa	15g
Bai Zi	Angelica dahurica	12g
Zi Su Ye	Perillae Folium	12g
Chen Pi	Citri Reticulatae Pericarpium	9g

Ban xia	Pinelliae Rhizoma	12g
Fu Ling	Poria	12g
Gan cao	Glycyrrhiza Uralensis	6g
Jie Geng	Platycodon grandiflorus (Jacq.)	9g
Hou Po	Mangnoliae Officinalis Cortex	9g

Comment

Huo Xiang Zheng Qi San is a famous Song Dynasty formula, designed for an unseasonable evil qi attacking the respiratory and digestive systems simultaneously. Manifested as a wind-cold exterior with dampness in the Middle Jiao interiorly. It combines antiviral herbs like Huo Xiang, Bai Zi, Zi Su Ye, together with Stomach harmonizing herbs like Chen Pi, Hou Po. Huo Xiang Zheng Qi San is applicable for Stomach flu, acute gastritis or acute gastroenteritis, H1N1, even COVID-19. Adopted as a patent formula in the national protocol, it became so popular that every family kept it as a home remedy. People call it Agastache Anti-Stomach Flu Powder.

Dampness predominate pattern:

Huo Po Xia Ling Tang

Huo Xiang	Agastache rugosa	15g
Xing Ren	Semen Armeniacae Amarum	12g
Yi Yi Ren	SemenCoicis	15g
Bai Dou Kou	Amomum cardamomum	9g
Dan Dou Shi	Sojae Semen Praeparatum	9g
Zhu Ling	Polyporus umbellatus	12g
Ze Xie	Alisma plantago-aquatica Linn	12g
Ban xia	Pinelliae Rhizoma	12g
Fu Ling	Poria	12g
Hou Po	Mangnoliae Officinalis Cortex	9g

Heat predominate pattern:

Gan Lu Xiao Du Dan (Sweet Dew Detoxify Decoction)

Huo Xiang	Agastache rugosa	15g
Bo He	Menta piperita	12g
Lian Qiao	Forsythia suspensa	15g
She Gan	Belamicandae Rhizome	12g
Huang Qin	Scutellaria baicalensis Georgi	15g
Chuan Bei Mu	Fritillaria cirrhosa D.Don	12g
Shi Chang Pu	Acorus tatarinowii	12g
Bai dou Kou	Amomum cardamomum	9g
Hua Shi	Talcum	15g
Mu Tong	Akebiae Caulis	15g
Yin Chen Hao	Artemisia capillaries	15g

Upper Jiao Xuan Bi Tang from *Detailed analysis on febrile diseases*

(Upper jiao disperse dampness heat Decoction)

Pi Pa Ye	Eriobotrya japonica Thunb	12g
She Gan	Belamicandae Rhizome	12g
Yu Jin	Curcumae Radix	15g
Tong Cao	Akebiae Caulis	15g
Dan Dou Chi	Sojae Semen Praeparatum	9g

Comment

Upper Jiao Xuan Bi Tang is a famous formula for Warm Dampness in the Upper Jiao, manifested as a stubborn fever, aversion to cold, fatigue with a heavy sensation, body aches, sore throat, cough heavily, nausea and vomiting, irritability.

Multiple studies have suggested that Yu Jin, the king herb of this formula (Curcumae Radix) which contains the active ingredient curcumin may be a potential prophylactic and treatment therapy for COVD-19. Since it has anti-viral and anti-inflammatory properties, Yu Jin also has the function to eliminate damp heat with it's aromatic characteristics, and is being used for warm dampness plague, this formula is a good example.

Evil qi hidden in MoYuan Pattern

Symptoms and signs: alternating fever and chills

Da Yuan Yin from the *Warm Plague Treatise* by Dr. Wu Youke

Open Mo Yuan Decoction

Bing Lang	Areca catechu L	15g
Cao Guo	Tsaoko Fructus	12g
Hou Po	Mangnoliae Officinalis Cortex	9g
Zhi Mu	Anemarrhenae Rhizoma	15g
Huang Qin	Scutellaria baicalensis Georgi	15g
Shao Yao	Paeonia Lactiflora Pall	12g
Gan Cao	Glycyrrhiza Uralensis	6g

Comment

Da Yuan Yin was created by Dr. Wu Youke, Ming Dynasty, considered the first medical man of the Wen Bing school. It is for warm diseases like flu or malaria. Mo Yuan manifests as alternating high fever and chills, headache, agitation, chest and abdominal fullness, nausea and vomiting. Red tongue with a thick, white and greasy coat, with white powder accumulated on the surface.

Three aromatic herbs Bing Lang, Cao Guo and Hou Po can eliminate turbid dampness, Huang Qin

Zhi Mu, Gan Cao can clear heat toxins, and Huang Qin has shown a strong inhibitory effect on COVID-19 virus in vitro, stronger than Lopinavir and Remdesivir. [13]. Gan Cao also showed the ability to inhibit replication of COVID-19 virus [14]. [15].

To explore the active compound of Da-Yuan-Yin for treatment of COVID-19, a study has been done. The methods were based on TCM's pharmacological platform (TCMSP). The chemical composition targets of Arecae Semen, Magnoliae Officinalis Cortex, Tsaoko Fructus, Anemarrhenae Rhizoma, Paeoniae Radix Alba, Scutellariae Radix, and Glycyrrhizae Radix et Rhizoma were screened.

The targets of corresponding gene were searched through UniProt, GeneCards databases, and then Cytoscape 3.2.1 was used to build compound-targets (genes) networks. The enrichment of gene ontology (GO) function analysis by DAVID and the pathway enrichment analysis by Kyoto Encyclopedia of Genes and Genomes (KEGG) were carried out, and the mechanism of its action was predicted.

Results are the compound-target network containing 141 compounds and 267 corresponding targets, and the key targets involved PTGS2, HSP90AA1, ESR1, AR, NOS2, etc. The function enrichment analysis of GO was 522 (P<0.05), of which there were 421 biological processes (BP) items, and 38 related items of cell composition (CC), and 63 molecular function (MF) items. There were 25 signal pathways (P<0.05) in the KEGG pathway enrichment screening, involving small cell Lung cancer, non-small cell Lung cancer and T cell receptor signaling pathways, etc. The results of molecular docking showed that the affinity of quercetin, kaempferol, baicalin and other core compounds was similar to recommended drugs recommended in the treatment of COVID-19.

The conclusion is that the active compounds in Da-Yuan-Yin may regulate multiple signaling pathways by binding angiotensin converting enzyme II (ACE2) and acting on targets such as PTGS2, HSP90AA1 and ESR1 to inhibit COVID-19.[16]

Middle Jiao Syndrome

Damp-heat with predominant heat

Signs and symptoms: high fever, red face, harsh breath, thirst, heavy sensation of the body with abdominal fullness, red tongue, yellowish, greasy coating, rapid and slippery pulse.

Bai Hu Jia Cang Zhu Tang (White Tiger add Cang Zhu Tang)

Shi Gao	Gypsum Fibrosum	24g
Zhi Mu	Anemarrhenae Rhizoma	15g
Stick rice	Oryza Sativa L	25g
Gan Cao	Glycyrrhiza Uralensis	6g
Cang Zhu	Atractylodes Lancea (Thunb.)	15g

Dampness heat in middle jiao:

Signs and symptoms: fever that is not relieved by sweating, thirst with no desire to drink, nausea, vomiting, abdominal fullness, yellowish and loose stool, yellow and scanty urine, red tongue with a thick, yellow and greasy coating, rapid and slippery pulse.

Wang Si Lian Po Yin (Dr.Wang's Lian Po Decoction)

Huang Lian	Coptis Salisb	12g
Zhi Zi	Gardenia Elli, nom, cons	15g
Dan dou Shi	Sojae Semen Praeparatum	9g
Hou Po	Mangnoliae Officinalis Cortex	9g
Shi Chang	Pu Acorus tatarinowii	12g
Ban Xia	Pinelliae Rhizoma	12g
Lu Geng	Phragmitis Rhizoma	20g

If the Middle Jiao and the Upper Jiao are simultaneously affected with damp-heat use

Xuan bi Tang from the *Detailed Analysis on Febrile Diseases*

Disperse Dampness Stagnation Decoction

Xing Ren	Semen Armeniacae Amarum	12g
Lian Qiao	Forsythia suspensa	15g
Zhi Zi	Gardenia Elli, nom, cons	15g
Yi Yi Ren	SemenCoicis	15g

Ban Xia	Pinelliae Rhizoma	12g
Chan Sha	Bombyx mori L	15g
Fang Ji	Stephaniae Tetrandrae Radix	15g
Hua Shi	Talcum	15g
Chi Xiao Dou	Vignae Semen	15g

For lingering dampness during the recovery period: fever decreased, still fullness in the Stomach and abdomen, hunger with no desire to eat, thin and greasy tongue coating.

Wu Ye Lu Geng Tang from the *Longitude and Latitude of Febrile diseases*

Dr. Xue's Five Leaf Lu Gen Decoction

Huo Xiang Ye	Agastache rugosa	15g
Bo He Ye	Menta piperita	12g
He Ye	Nelumbo nucifera Gaertn	15g
Pi Pa Ye	Eriobotrya japonica Thunb	12g
Pei Lan Ye	Eupatorium fortunei Turcz	15g
Lu Gen	Phragmitis Rhizoma	20g
Dong Gua Ren.	Benincasa hispida (Thunb.)	15g

Lower Jiao syndrome

(Damp heat obstructs orifice and Liver:

Signs and symptoms: convulsion, delirium, unclear mind, loss of consciousness, fever that is worse at night and better in the morning, there may be jaundice, red tongue with a yellow, greasy and thick coating, rapid and slippery pulse.

Cang Pu Yu Jin Tang

Shi Chang Pu	Acorus tatarinowii	12g
Yu Jin	Curcumae Radix	15g
Zhi Zi	Gardenia Elli, nom, cons	15g

Lian Qiao	Forsythia suspensa	15g
Ju Hua	Flos Chrysanthemi	12g
Hua Shi	Talcum	20g
Dan Zhu Ye	Lophatherum gracile	12g
Mu Dan Pi	Moutan Cortex	15g
Niu Bang Zi	Arctii Fructus	12g
Zhu Li	Bambusae Succus	15g
Sheng Jiang	Zingiber Officinale	12g

Damp heat transforming to fire and reaching the Ying and Blood level (DIC)

Signs and symptoms: High fever, irritability, bleeding (vomit with blood, stool with blood, cough with blood, urine with blood, bleeding under skin), crimson tongue.

Xiao Jiao Di huang Tang (Rhinoceros horn & rehmannia root cooling blood decoction)

Shui Niu Jiao	Cornu Bubali	12g
Shen Di Huang	Radix rehmanniae Recens	15g
Chi Shao Yao	Paeonia veitchii Lynch	15g
Mu Dan Pi	Moutan Cortex	15g

Damp heat obstructs lower Jiao, Kidney and Urinary Bladder dysfunction

Scanty urine or anuria, lower abdominal pain, thirst with no desire to drink, nausea, vomit, fever, unclear mind.

Fu Ling Pi Tang Detailed *analysis on febrile diseases*

Fu Ling Pi	Poria	12g
Yi Yi Ren	SemenCoicis	15g
Zhu Ling	Polyporus umbellatus	12g

Da Fu Pi	Arecae Pericarpium	15g
Tong Cao	Tetrapanax Medulla	12g
Dan Zhu Ye	Lophatherum gracile	12g

Kidney Yang Deficiency

Signs and Symptoms: edema on the face, limbs, pale and cold, fatigue, scanty urine, pale tongue and white coating, deep and weak pulse.

Zhen Wu Tang

(Hero Zhen Wu Decoction for Edema)

Fu Zi	Aconiti Lateralis Radix Praeparata	15g
Gan Jiang	Zingiber Officinale	12g
Bai Zhu	Atractylodes Macrocephala	12g
Fu Ling	Poria	12g
Bai Shao Yao	Paeonia Lactiflora	12g

Yang Qi collapse

Signs and symptoms: spontaneous cold sweat, pale complexion, harsh breath.

Du Sheng Tang (Single Ren Sheng Decoction)

| Ren Shen | Panax ginseng C.A.Mey | 15g |

After the Wen Bing School became established, together with the Shang Han School, TCM matured greatly in its treatment for epidemic diseases. Those theories turned out to be powerful tools of understanding, analysis and treatment for plagues including an understanding, analysis of COVID-19 aetiology, pathogenesis and treatment.

Reference

[1][2][3]. National Bureau of TCM. Chinese Protocol on COVID-19: 74.000 patients treated with Chinese Herbal Medicine, effective rate more than 90%. MedSci.cn 2020-3-24

[4]. Mechanism of preventing and treating COVID-19 with Traditional Chinese Medicine. Zhao Xia Etc. Journal of Nanjing University of Traditional Chinese Medicine. 2020.11.

[5][7][8]. Yellow Emperor's Inner Classic. Edited by Xu, Wenbing, published by People's publishing house.

[6]. Nan Jin.Yellow Emperor's Difficulty Questions.China Medicine and Pharma Publish House.

[7]. Lu Junxian etc.The development of research on anti-Flu virus effects of honeysuckle. Modern Chinese Medicine research and practice. 2018,20(6):25-27.

[8]. Zhou Z.etc. Honeysuckle-encoded atypical microRNA2911 directly targets influenza A viruses Cell Res.2015,25(1):39-49

[9]. Luo Xuan etc. Study on anti-virus H7N9 of Honeysuckle and Forsythia [j] modern Chinese Medicine.2016,36(2):75-78

[10] Nomura Effects of traditional Kamp drugs on influenza virus replication in vitro: suppression of viral protein synthesis by glycyrrhizae radix [J] Evid Based Complement Alternative Med.2019.:3230906.

[11]. Traditional Chinese medicine Lianhua Qingwen treating coronavirus disease 2019(COVID-19): Meta-analysis of randomized controlled trials. Mengjie Zeng etc.

Published: September 11, 2020. https://doi.org/10.1371/journal.pone.0238828

[12].Qinhai Ma et. The study on the treatment of Xuebijing injection (XBJ) in adults with severe or critical coronaVirus Disease 2019 and inhibitory effect of XBJ against SARS-Cov-2.www.ncbi.nlm.gov

[13]. Scutellaria baicalensis extract and baicalein inhibit replication of SARS-CoV-2 and its 3C-like protease in vitro MedSci. 2020-4-14

[14]. Glycyrrhizic Acid Exerts Inhibitory Activity against the Spike Protein of SARS-CoV- (2020《Phytomedicine》。

[15]. An artificial intelligence system reveals liquiritin inhibits SARSCoV-2 by mimicking type I interferon. bioRxiv

[16]. Exploring active compounds of Da-Yuan-Yin in treatment of COVID-19 based on network pharmacology and molecular docking method.Zong Yang etc. [J] Chinese Herbal Medicine. 2020, 51(4):836-844

Chapter Two

Preventive Treatment and Management of Covid-19

Preventive Treatment for COVID-19

People with certain underlying medical conditions are more likely to experience dangerous symptoms when infected with COVID-19. These include diabetes, severe obesity, high blood pressure, atherosclerosis, coronary disease, congestive Heart failure, hyperlipidemia, Kidney disease, asthma, chronic bronchitis, COPD, weakened immune system, cancers, and smokers.

In a study evaluating 1,099 laboratory-diagnosed patients with COVID-19 in China, COPD was detected in 1.1% patients. In a meta-analysis evaluating the incidence of underlying diseases in patients with COVID-19 requiring hospitalization, 0.95% of patients were found to have COPD (1). In another meta-analysis investigating the risk factors associated with patients with COVID-19, patients with COPD were found to have a 5.97-fold increased risk (2).

Therefore, it is important for those patients to preventively treat the potential susceptibility of infection, especially after exposure to Covid-19.

The occurrence, progress and recovery of Covid-19 is determined by a person's immune function. *Huang Di Nei Jing* says: "All evils of various seasons are harmful to people, they attack the body when it is vulnerable, and they should be defended anytime and everywhere. When one is completely free from wishes, ambitions, and distracting thought, indifferent to fame and gain, the True energy (Zhen Qi) will come in the wake of it. When one concentrates their spirit internally and keeps a sound mind, how can any illness occur? If there is no essence stored inside of the body in winter, humans will have warm, febrile diseases in the spring. No weak energy, no evils invading". Since then, TCM physicians focus on susceptibility related to the Lungs, Spleen, Kidney and immune function as well as physical constitution of patients.

A practitioner, Jiayan Yu (1585—1664) said: "The most important medicinals to take are the aromatic and supplementing herbs before Wen Bing, which prevents the Evils from invading the body. If the evils are already inside, the most important treatment is to strongly expel turbid evils. The Upper Jiao functions like a mist, if there are evils in it, lift them and expel them, and concurrently detoxify. The Middle Jiao functions like foam, if there are evils in it, transport & expel them, and concurrently detoxify. The Lower Jiao function is like a ditch, if there are evils in it, drain & expel them, and concurrently detoxify.

Preventively Treat for Underlying Respiratory Disorders and Immune disorders

The patients who have primary respiratory diseases and weakened immune systems tend to suffer from Spleen and Lung Qi deficiency and weak Wei Qi as root symptoms. The branch symptoms are the toxins of Covid-19 invading the body.

Yin deficiency with phlegm in the Lung

bThe patient who has primary Lung Yin deficiency or cancer patient has been treated by chemo/radiotherapy that injures the yin and is prone to get viral infections tend to experience heat invasion patterns. The Lung Yin tends to become scorched severely, resulting in fever, dry cough or cough with little sputum, even chronic cough.

Manifestations: typical symptoms of their primary Lung diseases or immune disorders, cough with sticky yellow phlegm, night sweats, low- grade fever, constipation, red tongue with peeled tongue coating, deep, thin and rapid pulse.

Treatment Strategy: nourish Lung Yin, eliminate damp and phlegm, prevent Covid-19.

Formula: Qing Zhao Jiu Fei Tang.

For prevention, add Jin Yin Hua, Qing Hao. For significant Lung Yin deficiency, add Bai He, Yu Zhu, or Sha Shen Mai Dong Tang to replace Qing Zhao Jiu Fei Tang. For Lung Qi and Yin deficiency, add Sheng Mai San. For severe phlegm, add Gua Lou, Lu Gen. For significant deficiency of the Lungs and Kidneys, Qing Zhao Jiu Fei Tang is replaced with Bai He Gu Jin Tang.

Acupuncture points: Lu9, St36, Ki3, St40, Ren22.

For preventing wind invasion, add Sj5, LI20. For significant Lung Yin deficiency, add UB23, SP6. For Lung Qi and Yin deficiency, add UB13, UB20.

Qi deficiency with damp phlegm accumulation in the Lungs

Patients who have primary diseases, such as chronic bronchitis, COPD, immune disorders with Lung Qi deficiency are susceptible to flu virus and other viral infections that can easily injure the Qi or Yang and lead to phlegm accumulating in the Lungs.

Manifestations: all typical signs and symptoms from the patient's primary disease will be present, feeble cough, dyspnea, shortness of breath, fatigue and weak voice, spontaneous sweating, frequently suffering cold or flu, pale tongue with white pulse, deep and weak pulse.

Treatment strategy: supplement Lung Qi, strengthen the exterior, eliminate dampness, resolve phlegm and prevent infection.

Formula: Yu Ping Feng San, add Huo Xiang, Zi Su Ye.

For prevention, add Cao Guo, Sha Ren. For significant Qi deficiency, add Ren Shen, Wu Wei Zi. For significant phlegm, add Chen Pi, Ban Xia.

Acupuncture points: LI20, LU5, ST36, UB20, REN12.

For significant damp phlegm, add SP9, ST40. For significant Qi deficiency, add REN6, SP6 with moxa. For Qi deficiency of the Lung and Kidney, add UB13, UB23, DU4.

Heart blood stasis

The patient who has primary Heart disorders due to Qi stagnation and blood stasis blocking the Heart meridian, which slows down the Qi production of Lung, leads to the patient being susceptible to the virus. Meanwhile, the disease can cause more blood stagnation when the patient suffers from the Covid-19, which makes the disease very complicated.

Manifestations: The symptoms of primary cardiovascular disorders, chest stiffness, anxiety, irritability, palpitations, insomnia, purple tongue with watery coating, choppy pulse.

Treatment Strategy: invigorate blood, open meridian and prevent infection

Formula: Xue Fu Zhu Yu Tang, Liu Ji Lu, Hu Zhang.

For chest pain, add Dan Shen, Yu Jin. For anxiety, irritability and insomnia, add Suan Zao Ren, Wu Wei Zi. For hypercholesterolemia, add Hong Mi, Jiao Shan Zha. For preventing infection of the virus, add Jang Huang, Zi Ju Hua.

Acupuncture points: PC6, HT7, UB15, UB17.

For chest pain, add Ren14, PC7. For anxiety, irritability and insomnia, add Anmian, Ear HT, Ear Shen Men. For hypercholesterolemia, add ST40, SP10, ST36.

Heart Qi and Yin deficiency

Patients with primary cardiac and respiratory disorders, and patients with chronic Heart Qi and Yin deficiency will have a higher susceptibility to infection of Covid-19.

Manifestations: The symptoms of primary cardiovascular disorders will be present, palpitations, fatigue, insomnia, dreams, poor memory, profuse sweating, small and pale tongue with less coating, deep and weak rapid pulse.

Treatment Strategy: supplement Qi and Yin of the Heart and prevent viruses.

Formula: Sheng Mai San and Dan Shen Yin.

For significant Qi and Yin deficiency, add Huang Qi and Bai He. For significant insomnia, dreams a lot, add Suan Zao Ren, Bai Zi Ren.

Acupuncture Points: ST36, UB15, UB20, PC6.

For significant Qi and Yin deficiency, add UB23, Rer14. For significant insomnia, excessive dreaming, add Yin Tang, Ear Shen Men.

Heart Yang deficiency

Most of the patients who have primary Heart disorders, chronic respiratory disorders with Qi and Yin deficiency of Heart, will have a higher potential for Covid-19 infection. The toxin of Covid-19 tends to injure the Heart.

Manifestations: All typical symptoms of primary cardiovascular disorders, perhaps even congestive Heart failure, severe palpitations, unable to lie flat, bilateral lower leg edema, cold extremities, pale and swollen tongue with watery coating, deep weak pulse.

Treatment Strategy: Warm the Heart Yang, supplement Heart Qi and prevent virus.

Formula: Shen Fu Hong Ting Tang.

In the formula, Hong Shen is for supplementing the Heart Qi, Fu Zi warms Heart Yang, Hong Hua invigorates the blood and Ting Li Zi purges water retention from the Lungs. For significant edema, add Wu Ling San (Poria Five Powder). For significant cold extremities, add Rou Gui, Gan Jiang.

Acupuncture Points: Ren8, Ren17, PC6, HT7, ST36.

Add moxa at Ren8. For significant edema, add SJ5, UB40. For significant cold extremities, add DU4 with moxa.

Damp-heat accumulation in the Spleen and Stomach

Many people have primary digestive disorders, such as gastritis and peptic ulcers. The physical constitution of damp-heat determines the patient's vulnerability to Covid-19 infection. Covid-19 has many characteristics of dampness and heat, both which damages the Spleen and Stomach which will lead to a worsening of their primary disorder.

Manifestations: all symptoms of their primary disorder will be present, such as gastritis and peptic ulcers. They also have Stomachache, acid regurgitation, abdominal bloating, bad breath, heavy body, red tongue with thick yellow greasy coating, and sluggish pulse.

Treatment strategies: clear heat, eliminate dampness of the Spleen and Stomach, prevent the virus.

Formula: Lian Po Yin (Coptis and Magnolia Decoction).

For Stomachache, add Yan Hu Suo, Zhi Shi. For acid regurgitation, add Duan Long Gu and Duan Mu Li. For significant heat, add Chong Lou and Hu Zhang.

Acupuncture points: Ren12, ST25, SP9, ST36.

For Stomachache, add ST34, ST21. For abdominal bloating, add LIV13, ST38. For acid regurgitation, add PC6, GB34. For significant heat, add ST44, or bleed Er Jian.

Spleen Qi deficiency with damp accumulation

Most of these patients have primary digestive disorders, such as chronic gastritis, chronic peptic ulcers and chronic indigestion. All of those disorders lead to damp pathogen diseases, such as Covid-19.

Manifestations: all symptoms of their primary digestive disorder are present, diarrhea, poor appetite, tasteless, fatigue, pale and swollen tongue with white greasy coating, deep weak pulse.

Treatment strategies: supplement Spleen Qi, eliminate dampness and prevent viruses.

Formula: Liu Jun Zi Tang (Six Gentlemen Decoction)

For patients who have dampness greater than heat, heaviness in the body, fullness of chest and loss of taste choose the Huo Po Xia Ling Tang (Patchouli, Magnolia, pinellia and Poria Decoction). For diarrhea, add Yi Yi Ren, Shan Yao. For loss of taste, add Huo Xiang, Pei Lan. To prevent infection, add Cao Guo, Bai Dou Kou.

Acupuncture points: ST36, SP9, REN12, SP6.

For severe diarrhea, add SP4, UB20. Add moxa at ST36, REN12. For tastelessness, add REN23, Ear Shen Men.

Liver Qi stagnation: When patients have primary disorders that are relative to Liver and Gallbladder diseases in TCM, such as hypertension, depression, hepatitis they are also easily complicated with Liver Qi stagnation during the pandemic, triggering the pandemic pathogen that easily attacks the patient.

Manifestations: The patients have primary symptoms of hypertension, depression, and hepatitis. Also stress, hypochondriac pain, short temper, acid regurgitation, fullness of abdomen and poor appetite, irregular period, thin white coating and wiry pulse.

Treatment strategies: Soothe Liver, strengthen Spleen and prevent the virus.

Formula: Jia Wei Xiao Yao San (Free and Easy Plus)

For hypochondria pain, add Yu Jin, Fo Shou. For significant depression, add He Huan Pi, Ye Jiao Teng. For short temper and acid regurgitation, add Long Gu, Mu Li. For significant Qi stagnation turning to heat, add Da Qing Ye, Yin Chen.

Acupuncture points: LIV3, LI4, SP4, REN12.

For hypochondria pain, add LIV13. For significant depression, add Yintang, Ear Shen Men. For short temper and acid regurgitation, add GB34, GB41. For significant Qi stagnation turning to heat, add ST44.

Damp-heat of Liver and Gallbladder

When patients have primary disorders such as hepatitis, cholecystitis due to damp-heat of Liver and Gallbladder, their Livers are easily injured by Covid-19 infection.

Manifestations: The patients have primary symptoms of hepatitis, cholecystitis, hypertension, and depression. They may also have rib-side fullness and pain, jaundice, heavy sensation of the body, poor appetite, red tongue with thick yellow greasy coating, wiry pulse.

Treatment strategies: clear heat and eliminate dampness of Liver and Gallbladder, prevent the virus.

Formula: Yin Chen Wu Ling San (Artemisiae scopariae Five Ling powder)

For a heavy sensation of the body, add Huo Xiang, Zi Su Ye. For increased appetite, add Bai Bian Dou, Shan Yao. To prevent viral infection, add Qing Hao, Sha Ren.

Acupuncture points: LIV3, GB34, SJ5, SP9.

For a heavy body sensation, add Si Shen Chong, ST40. For increased appetite, add Ren12, ST36.

Hyperactivity of Liver Yang with Yin deficiency

When patients have primary disorders such as hypertension due to hyperactivity of Liver Yang with Yin deficiency, their Liver Yin can be further injured by Covid-19.

Manifestations: The patients have primary symptoms of hypertension, headache, dizziness, bad temper, irritability, reddish eyes, red tongue with yellow coating, wiry rapid pulse.

Treatment strategies: calm the Liver and sedate Yang, prevent the virus.

Formula: Tian Ma Gou Teng Yin (Gastrodia-Uncaria Decoction).

For a significant headache, add Chuan Xiong, Ju Hua. For bad temper and irritability, add Long Gu and Mu Li.

Acupuncture points: GB20, LIV3, GB41, LI11.

For a significant headache, add local points. For bad temper and irritability, add Yintang, bleed the ear hypertension point and ear Shenmen.

Kidney Yin deficiency

When patients have primary disorders such as chronic nephritis, or Xiao Ke due to Kidney Yin deficiency, their Kidneys will be further damaged by Covid-19.

Manifestations: The patients have symptoms of primary chronic nephritis, Xiao Ke, low back and knee pain, night urine, hot sensation with night sweating, red tongue with dry mouth, thin and rapid pulse.

Treatment strategies: Nourish Kidney Yin, clear heat, prevent the virus.

Formula: Zhi Bai Di Huang Wan (Anemarrhena-Phellodendron-Rehmannia Pill)

For significant thirst, add Tian Hua Fen, Xuan Shen. For low back and knee pain, add Sang Ji Sheng, and Niu Xi. For hot sensation with night sweating, add Qing Hao, Bai He, E Jia.

Acupuncture points: UB23, KI3, Ren3, SP6.

For Xiao Ke, add Wei Wan Xia Shu, KI6. For low back and knee pain, add DU4, Yaoyan. For hot sensations with night sweating, add HT7.

Kidney Yang deficiency

When patients have severe Lung, Heart, Spleen and Kidney primary disorders, they gradually damage Kidney Yang. These patients are prone to be invaded by the exterior pathogens including Covid-19. Their Kidneys are further damaged by Covid-19 infection.

Manifestations: The patients have symptoms of primary disorders, edema, profuse nocturia, coldness in the low back and knee pain, cold extremities, pale swollen with watery coating, deep weak and slow pulse.

Treatment strategies: warm and supplement Kidney Yang, prevent the virus.

Formula: Zhen Wu Tang (True Warrior Decoction)

For significant edema, add Wu Ling San (Five Poria Powder). For significant cold extremities, add Gui Zhi and Ren Shen. For viral prevention, add Huang Qi and Cao Guo.

Acupuncture points: DU4, Ren8, ST36, DU20.

For significant edema, add SP9, UB40. For significant cold extremities, add moxa at DU4, REN8.

Reference:

1.Emami A, Javanmardi F, Pirbonyeh N, Akbari A. Prevalence of underlying disease in hospitalized patients with COVID-19: A systematic review and meta-analysis. *Arch Acad Emerg Med.* 8: e35. 202.

2.Wang B, Li R, Lu Z, Huang Y. Does comorbidity increase the risk of patients with COVID-19: evidence from meta-analysis. *Aging (Albany NY)* 2020; 12:6049–57. doi: 10.18632/aging.103000.

TCM Preventive Management of COVID-19

If COVID-19 is spreading in your community, stay safe by taking some simple precautions, such as physical distancing, wearing a mask, keeping rooms well ventilated, avoiding crowds, cleaning your hands, and coughing into a bent elbow or tissue. Check local advice where you live and work.

You also find out more about the WHO's recommendations for getting vaccinated on our public advice page on COVID-19 vaccines.

How to Protect Yourself & Others?

U.S CDC recommends the following to prevent COVID-19 (https://www. cdc.gov/coronavirus/2019-ncov/prevent-getting-sick/index.html.)

- Wear a mask that covers your nose and mouth to help protect yourself and others.
- Stay 6 feet apart from others who don't live with you.
- Get a COVID-19 vaccine when it is available to you.
- Avoid crowds and poorly ventilated indoor spaces.
- Wash your hands often with soap and water. Use hand sanitizer if soap and water aren't available.

TCM also has measures for preventing pandemics. We will introduce the common preventive ways that have been used since ancient times:

Nasal care during a pandemic

These measures help to reduce the incidence of pandemic.

- Knead LI 20 with your finger five minutes, once every day. (Author's experience)
- Put a small piece of fresh garlic near the nose, during sleep, once a day (Yi Fang Kao. Investigations of Medical Formulas.1586)
- Put Zi Cao Oil, one drop with cotton swab near the nose before going to bed. Once every night. (Author's experience)
- To prepare Zi Cao Oil, put 30g of Zi Cao in 60 ml sesame oil and soak the Zi Cao in the oil for two weeks.
- To induce sneezing, put a cotton swab inside the nose until sneezing. Do this once in the morning and once before going to bed. (Wan Shi Ji Shi Liang Fang. Wan's Fine formulas of Aiding Life.1609).

Tong Qi San (Open Qi Powder) Inducing Sneeze: Touch a little of Tong Qi San with cotton swab and place it inside the nose to induce sneezing, do this three times per day. (Zha Bing Yuan Liu Xi Zhu. Wondrous Lantern for Peering into the Origin and Development of Miscellaneous Diseases. 1717-1776)

Tong Qi San: Yan Hu Suo 1.5g, Zhao Jiao 3g, Bai Shao3g, Li Lu 1g. Burn all of the herbs to ashes to make powder.

Eyes management during pandemic

- Yu Xing Cao Eye Drops (Patent remedy): use three times per day. (Author's experience).
- Ren Ma Ping An San: Bing Pian, She Xiang, Xiong Huang (Fei), Zhu Sha (Fei), each1.5g, Mang Xiao 3g. made them as powder. Put a little at UB1. (Yan Fang Xing Bian. Experience Formulas New compiled. 1875)

Oral management during pandemic

- Drink liquor: drink a small cup of liquor and wash the throat before and after going out during a pandemic (Jing Yan Shen Fang. Experienced and Effective Formulas. Qing Dynasty)
- Wash mouth with Herbal toothpaste:

Put Ku Shen on the toothpaste and brush the teeth. (Xiang Pu. Fragrant Formulas. 960-1127).

Put Song Zhi and Fu Ling on the toothpaste and brush the teeth. (Xiang Pu. Fragrant Formulas. 960-1127).

Put Huo Xiang and Pei Lan on the toothpaste, and brush the teeth. (Author's experience).

Body Management during pandemic

- Acupuncture for prevention: Please refer to the Preventive treatment of COVID-19.

Puncture LI20, ST36, LU11, GB20.

- Herbal Bath

Shi Qi Zhang Yi Yu Fang (Epidemic and Pandemic Washing Formula): Tao Zhi (Branches of Peach tree) 1000g, Bai Zhi (Radix Angelicae Dahuricae) 100g, Ce Bai Ye (Cacumen Platycladi) 500g. Grind all ingredients into powder and put 300g into hot water. Then take a bath with herbal water every day (Pu Ji Fang. Formulas of Universal Benefit. 1132).

Bi Wen Fang (Preventing Pandemic Formula): Chuan Xiong, Cang Zhu, Bai Zhi, Ding Xiang each have the same dosage, boil them together. Take a bath with the herb formula three times. Promote slight sweating. (Song Feng Shuo Yi. Songfeng on Pandemic. 1782)

- Powdering the body: Powdering the body is an ancient therapy that puts the herbal powders on the body to treat or prevent diseases.

Chi San Fang (Red powder formula): Mu Dan Pi 1.5g, Zao Jiao1.5g, Xi Xin1g, Gan Jiang 1g, Fu Zi 1g, Rou Gui 1g, Zhen Zhu Mu1.8g, grind them all into powder. Put the powder on the body once a day. (Zhou Hou Bie Ji Fang. Emergency Formula to Keep Up One's Sleeve. 341)

- Herbal Smoke Air Therapy: Burned herbs can be used for disinfecting the air.

Bi Wen San (Prevent Pandemic Powder): Put Ru Xiang, Mo Yao, Cang Zhu, Xi Xin, Chuan Xiong, Gan Cao, Da Zao all together, and burn them in the room.

Ai Pu Gua Fang: Ai Ye 50g, Shi Chang Pu 50g. Hang the herbs at the front door of the house.

Boiling Vinegar: put 30 ml of vinegar in a small pot and cook on low heat for about one hour, once per day. (Author's experience)

- Herbal Pouch Therapy: Herbs can be worn for disinfection and prevention of pandemic. The herbs usually are aromatic.

Zhi He Xiang Nang (Fragrant Bag): 10g of Cang Zhu, Huo Xiang, Bai Zhi and Bo He are made into powder, and placed in a small bag. The patient wears it on the chest.

- Taking herbs for prevention: please refer to the Preventive treatment of COVID-19 section.

Chapter Three

TCM Treatment during Covid-19

Etiology, Pathogenesis and Treatment of COVID-19 according to TCM

In order to offer an effective treatment, we have done an etiology and pathogenesis analysis of COVID-19 within the framework of Traditional Chinese Medicine. As Dr. Sun Si Miao said "If one wants treatment for disease, they must first look for the causes, and the pathological changes within the symptoms and signs (*Thousand gold worth formulas. Diagnosis on manifestation*) The general view within the Chinese Medicine community at present is that the broad meaning of Shang Han includes febrile diseases (Pyreticosis) or infectious diseases. The *Yellow Emperor Inner Classic* states clearly "Nowadays febrile diseases all belong to Shang Han". The *Medical Difficulty questions No.58* pointed out further "There are five kinds of Shang Han, induced by wind, coldness, warm-dampness, heat, and by Wen Bing.

When a pathogen is more contagious it is called Wen Bing. Later generations began with Dr.Wang Menying, Qing Dynasty. He classified the narrow meaning of Shang Han into Wen Bing, he considered cold and heat as one integration, cold as latitude and heat as longitude. His book was named Wen *Bing latitude and longitude*. Dr.Wu Jutong, Qing Dynasty, listed nine kinds of Wen Bing. Wen Bing includes wind warmth, warmth heat, warm plague, warm toxin, summer heat, damp warmth, autumn dryness, winter warmth, and warm malaria. Under the principle of syndrome differentiation to identify etiology, TCM methods of Shang Han, Six Meridian Syndrome Differentiation, Wen Bing, Wei Qi Ying Xue Differentiation and San Jiao Syndrome Differentiation have been applied to make an analysis on Covid-19 symptoms and signs based on documents reported. We discovered that Covid-19 has apparent characteristics of Turbid Dampness. After an analysis, we have reached an initial conclusion that Covid-19 belongs to the Damp-warmth category.

COVID-19 has the obvious characteristics of turbid dampness, which is determined by the local natural climate, geography and diets as well as other factors. *The Yellow Emperor Inner Classic* said that heaven and earth generate plagues. The onset of COVID-19 is closely related with global warming, global economic integration, increasing urbanization, frequent population mobility, and population concentration etc. *The Yellow Emperor Inner Classic, Plain Questions* said " If seasonal dampness is not eliminated, people will become sick from plagues. Dr.Wu Jutong explained in more detail "When warm plagues are epidemic, they contain turbid dampness, every family gets sick with the same symptoms, like soldiers in an army". Dr.Wei Yiling, Yuan Dynasty, called it Damp plague and described "Too much rain in the autumn will cause (winter) damp plague, manifesting as alternating chills and fever, damage to the Lung Qi resulting in stormy-like cough, nausea, vomiting, macula on the skin, cough, wheezing, shortness of breath, and it is named Damp-warm plague. This description is very close to the manifestations of COVID-19.

Take the city of Wuhan in HuBei province, China as an example, it was the first place where COVID-19 was discovered, the question is why Wu Han?

Natural climate factors

Hubei Province has a subtropical monsoon climate. It is cloudy and humid all year long. In the summer it is intensely hot and humid. This heat can be stored in the body and is difficult to clear. During the winter, people are prone to get sick from hidden summer heat and catch severe colds. The humidity makes it feel like the coldness penetrates to the bone. In

Spring people are prone to get warm disease patterns, haze is serious due to vigorous industry, UV radiation disinfection is poor because of year-round cloudy weather, making it easier to spread disease. Records show an unusually cold and rainy winter since December 2019, that easily bring dampness

Geographical factors

Hubei is known as the place of a thousand lakes and is surrounded on three sides by mountains. Wuhan is made of three towns along two large rivers, a quarter of the surface of the province is water. Annual rainfall is 1269 mm, relative humidity can be up to 75%-90%, most of the landscape are plains, lakes, and hills, with poor air flow. Wuhan is one of four of the hottest cities in China. Hubei, like the neighboring provinces of Guangdong, Guangxi and Hunan, is a very humid place. Traditionally, epidemic diseases thrive in this climate.

Social factors

Wuhan is known as China's geographical, economic and transportation hub, nine provinces have access, and the population is highly dense. A highly urbanized mega city, it is one of the world's most important industrial chain cities. It is the country's most important industrial base, high-tech base, with a population of 11 million people, college students alone comprise almost 1 million. The population density of 120,000 people/square kilometers (New York 28,000, San Francisco 17,000/square mile), GDP growth and net inflow of young people is the country's second (45 percent are young people, more active mobile population), makes it easy for people to be in constant contact with one another. Local food tends to be very spicy and fatty. The people are supposed to be the smartest and the easiest to become stressed. All of those result in endogenetic damp-heat patterns. Dr. Xue Shengbai, Qing Dynasty, said "Tai Yin (Spleen) internal injury leads to damp fluid gathering, which interacts together with exterior evils and then damp heat plague happens".

(1). Sticky and contagious, highly contagious. The basic reproductive rate (*R*0) of Covid-19 is 1.8-3.6 compared with influenza is 1.8-1.9(https://www.ncbi.nlm.nih.gov/pmc/articles/PMC7333991/)

(2). Heavy cloudy turbid, fever but hot not radiate, worse at daytime, sweating sticky clothes, choking coughing, breathing harsh, tightness and suffocate on chest like drowning, worse with movement, sticky sputum, thirst but no desire of drinking, nausea and vomiting, diarrhea.

(3). Headache, body and joints pain with heavy sensation, fatigue, poor react, lazy to talk, clear orifices are blocked red eyes, smelling, tasting and hearing are decreased significantly, seemingly normal by looking.

(4). Tongue coat thick and moisture, can see miliaria alba on skin.

(5). More fake negative and asymptomatic cases, many asymptomatic cases, even break through cases after vaccination.

(6). Pandemic all over the world, all year long. lingering, may test positive again after cured and test negative.

Concurrently COVID-19 has the characteristics of Damp Heat in the Three Jiao. Initially it attacks the Upper Jiao (Lungs) with fever, cough, and wheezing (89.6%) (ARDS). Then we may see Middle Jiao (Spleen, Stomach) trapped with dampness causing vomiting and diarrhea (30%). And it may diffuse to all three Jiao, blinding the upper Heart orifice leading to confusion (45%), loss of smell, taste and hearing. While damage to the lower jiao (Liver, Kidney), Kidney damage occurs in 8-12% of cases, as well as decreased reproductive function. Secondly, COVID-19 has the common characteristics of Wen Bing (warm plague). First of all it attacks the Lungs (95.6% onset with pneumonia change in X-ray), especially B1.617. Pneumonia may happen very early on, and a deteriorating condition within 8-10 hours. Serious cases (18-20%) will transform into heat-fire toxin, septicemia triggering a cytokine storm. This adversely transforms to the Pericardium (confuse mind 45.6%, 50% of ICU patients with myocarditis, pericarditis, Heart functional failure). This may get into the Ying level and the Blood level leading to disseminated intravenous coagulation (DIC), blood clotting, shock and multiple organ failure, death comes soon afterwards.

Profuse small vessel vasculitis due to heat at ying and blood may cause Kawasaki like illness in children (Pediatric inflammatory multisystem syndrome (PIMS). PIMS manifestes on the tongue as dark red, crimson red or purple dark, which looks like black waxberry.

In a closed environment with poor ventilation or high humidity, disease patterns will trend higher. Cruise ships, warships such as aircraft carriers, submarines, hospital ICU, prisons, office buildings, senior facilities, slaughterhouses. The Diamond Princess cruise ship and the Charles de Gaulle aircraft carrier have become experimental models.

It is now known that the aerosol state of the new coronavirus' survival time, air transmission distance, and transmission height are much more than expected. We don't even know all the details yet. Studies indicate that this new coronavirus' survival time is 240 minutes when the temperature is 10-15 centigrade (50 F), 2-30 minutes when 25 degrees centigrade (77 F), but the survival time in 24 hours of a respiratory droplet at room temperature, people continue to argue about this point. Surely it is a typical bio-aerosol, in which it may contain viral, bacteria, fungal, or pollen etc. It is a very important pathologic factor from the TCM perspective. In southern China where the climate is hot and humid, epidemics often happen. Humid, damp heat is the basis of the formation of epidemics. Epidemics are the most contagious and toxic diseases. TCM noticed this phenomenon very early on, it found that it can be in limited, small areas or it can be ubiquitous in widespread geographical areas. Both situations are high-risk, and evacuation must be mandatory, the area needs to be locked down.

Dr. Zhang Jingyue had lined out the city closure measures: no travel abroad, as well as disallowing foreigners into the state. He pointed out the importance of staying home because when people stay home, they rest. Travellers are often tired, 80-90% of travellers will become infected when visiting an infectious zone. There are epidemics that occur in all four seasons. It can manifest as cold patterns, heat patterns, mental disorders, or malaria-like epidemics. They can be human-to-human, can be animals passed on to people (snakes, birds, pets, peacock, bees, chickens and ducks, earthworm etc.), Zhang Zhongjing warned not to eat beaver meat, Li Shizhen warned about eating bats, epidemics can even be from plant to people (cinnamon flowers, chrysanthemums, etc.)

It has been proven that air transmission of the new coronavirus in an aerosol state is one of the most important routes of transmission other than spitting. This is especially true through nasal inhalation.The nasal mucous membrane has a high expression Ace2, and some scholars speculate that is the main way it enters the body. In Chinese Medicine, only Damp plague can explain the highly pathogenic infectiousness and severity of the new coronavirus, therefore isolating patients and quarantine are the most important anti-miasma measures. Statistics have shown that the ICU hospitalization rate in Hubei Province is significantly higher than in the rest of China: 21.9% to 0.5% (p<0.5% 001), and Covid-19's death rate in Hubei province is also significantly higher than in non-Hubei area: 10.4% to 0.6% (p<0.001), we speculate that is mainly due to local miasma which is a bio- aerosol status route.

Moreover, the new coronavirus has the characteristics of a plague pandemic. From December 2019 to date, the new coronavirus pneumonia epidemic found in Wuhan City, Hubei Province, China, has spread worldwide, becoming the world's largest public health crisis in a hundred years since the 1918 Spanish pandemic. So far (May.14, 2021), 1.61378940 million people have been confirmed worldwide, with 3.347190 million deaths. All 6 continents and more than 221 countries are involved. India is being stricken severely, Europe and Northern America are experiencing a third wave. We are all experiencing one of the most severe epidemics in modern time, even though there are vaccines. It seems this will not end by 2022, many speculate that it may come yearly like flu, and that the world's economy will not recover by 2025. Summarizing all of the above, COVID-19 belongs to the category of warm dampness. The cause is dampness and warm evil. The characteristics of an epidemic, even pandemic, can be defined as a warm dampness plague in TCM. As said in Ye Tianshi's *Medical case.Warm plague study* "one person affected means warm dampness, in an area many affected means warm damp plague". Dr.Yu Chang, Qing Dynasty also said "Warm dampness includes epidemic conditions, when warm dampness gets worse, then everyone gets it no matter older or younger with similar symptoms, that is called a warm and damp plague".

The study of Chinese Medicine on aetiology and pathology of COVID-19 is in the preliminary exploratory stage, and the source of information on symptomological evidence in this paper is mainly based on:

World Health Organization 10,000 case characteristics report.

Zhong Nanshan team 3,000 cases report, Lancet report characteristic analysis study.

China Health Care Commission organization pathology anatomy report.

Beijing TCM Hospital, Chinese Medicine Research Institute, Wuhan Jinyintan Hospital, Wuhan Central Hospital, Guangdong Provincial Hospital and Shenzhen Central Hospital related symptoms reports

The methods of analyzing the above information are Shang Han Six Meridian Syndrome differentiation, Wen Bing, Wei Qi Ying Xue Syndrome Differentiation, Damp Heat Three Jiao differentiation combined with eight principal differentiation, and Zang Fu syndrome differentiation. Through comprehensive analysis, we try to find out all aspects of Chinese Medicine characteristics of COVID-19, understand its essence, then establish principles of treatment, and treatment methods, and prescriptions selection.

Shang Han School Perspective

COVID-19 follows the law of the Six Stages of transmission. Infection begins in the three-yang, Tai Yang, Shao Yang, Yang Ming, and then moves to the three Yin stages, Tai Yin, Jue Yin, Shao Yin. Development can be sequential from exterior to interior, or it may directly attack the interior from the beginning. Oftentimes the three yang stages are struck simultaneously, and there may be Yang and Yin stages that are co-affected.

The three yang stages are relatively less severe, while the three yin stages are advanced stages, even deadly. The three yang stages are more in the Qi level, the three yin stages, especially Jue Yin, correspond to the Blood level. Eventually if the disease enters into the Shao Yin stage, the patient is then critical and many will die.

Wen Bing School Perspective

COVID-19 also follows the laws of Wei Qi Ying Xue transmission. The initial Wei level directly attacks the Lung. Many people will recover quickly if the pathogen remains at this level. In some patients the evil qi will transforms into a fire toxin, transmitting adversely into the Pericardium, burning body fluids, then entering into the Ying and Blood level causing septicaemia, leading to the cytokine storm syndrome, and possibly combined with disseminated intravascular coagulation (DIC). Then the patient will experience secondary shock, multi-organ failure, putting them in a critical condition.

Three Jiao Perspective

COVID-19 follows the law of Three Jiao transmission. First it attacks the Upper Jiao (Lung), many combine with the Middle Jiao (Spleen and Stomach), and the worst cases may diffuse between all three Jiao, blinding the Pericardium, and at the Lower Jiao leading to Liver and Kidney damage. At this point the patient is considered critical.

In summary, we think of COVID-19 pathogenesis is caused by Warm Dampness plague, often starting its attack in the Upper Jiao, hidden in the intrapleural-diaphragmatic space. The Lung Qi is blocked, it fails to disperse and descend. Then it transforms into interior heat, phlegm fluid obstruction, Qi and Blood stagnation, causing tissue damage and blood decay, finally developing into Lung abscess.

In younger stronger persons with strong vital qi, or people who are treated promptly and properly, while the evil qi is comparative weak and there is good prognosis, even though dampness may linger, phlegm and blood stagnation may occur, it is called Desirable Syndrome.

In elderly or weak people, those who have poor constitutions, ones who are not treated promptly or properly the evil qi is comparatively strong and often transforms into fire toxin. The pathogen frequently invades deeper into the Ying and Blood levels and pervades the three Jiao. Oftentimes

causing Yang Ming Fu Syndrome (Toxic paralytic intestinal obstruction syndrome), Invade the Chest Syndrome (Myocarditis, Pericarditis) , Chest binding syndrome (Pleuritis) , or water retention (Pleural Effusion). Liver and Kidney damage can result in Obstruction Syndrome

Brain damage, and even prolapsed syndrome (Shock). In these cases, the prognosis is poor sometimes critical and the person may die. Just like Dr.Wu Jutong recorded in *Detailed analysis of Warm plague.Upper Jiao* there are many ways people may die from Wen Bing, but principally no more than those five. Initially Lung Qi exhaustion (Respiratory failure), secondly, Obstruction Syndrome interiorly (Brain damage), Exteriorly Prolapsed Syndrome (Shock), the third is Yang Ming Fu syndrome (Toxic paralytic intestinal obstruction), the fourth is Spleen dampness steaming the Liver causing jaundice, severe jaundice blocked orifice (Kernicterus) leading to death. The fifth is Lower Jiao orifice blocked by turbid dampness causing death (Kidney functional failure), or damage to the Kidney essence.

COVID-19 is supposed to be located mainly in the Lung and Spleen, but all five inner organs may be involved. Qi and Blood may both be injured; the disease may pervade all three Jiao. Turbid dampness, phlegm fluids, heat in the blood and blood stagnation all predominate. The syndrome differentiation is assumed to be one of excess with deficiency.

Severe deficiency can lead to prolapsed syndrome while extreme excess may lead to obstruction syndrome. During the recovery period, vital Qi is weak and evil Qi lingers. Both vital Qi and evil Qi are weak, there may be blood stagnation with phlegm, manifesting as pulmonary fibrosis (PF). The water and dampness remain sticky and linger together. Covid tests will continue to show positive.

Covid-19 Etiology and pathogenesis

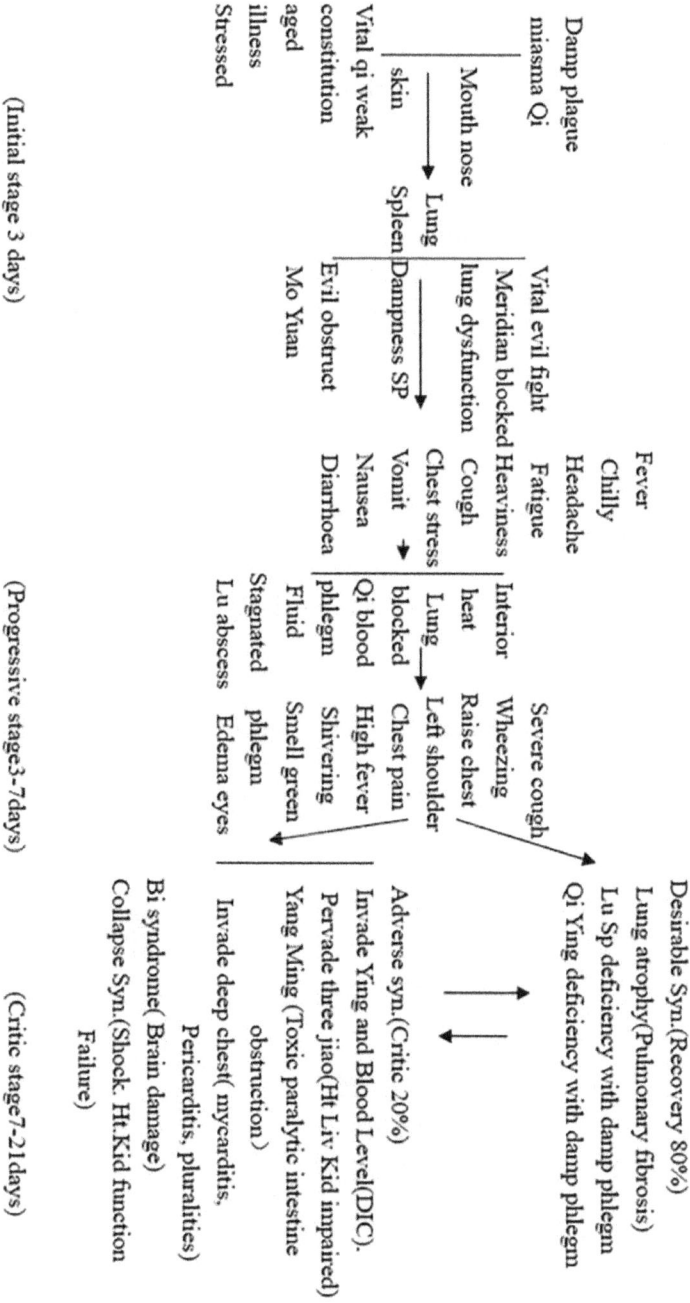

Damp plague miasma Qi

Vital qi weak
constitution
aged
illness
Stressed

— skin
— Mouth nose

Spleen Dampness SP
Lung

Evil obstruct
Mo Yuan

Vital evil fight
Meridian blocked lung dysfunction

Fever
Chilly
Headache
Fatigue

Heaviness
Cough
Chest stress

Vomit
Nausea
Diarrhoea

Interior heat
Lung blocked
Lung → Raise chest

blocked
Qi blood
phlegm
Fluid
Stagnated phlegm
Lu abscess

Wheezing
Severe cough

Chest pain
High fever
Shivering
Smell green
Edema eyes

Desirable Syn.(Recovery 80%)
Lung atrophy(Pulmonary fibrosis)
Lu Sp deficiency with damp phlegm
Qi Ying deficiency with damp phlegm

Adverse syn.(Critic 20%)
Invade Ying and Blood Level(DIC).
Pervade three jiao(Ht Liv Kid impaired)
Yang Ming (Toxic paralytic intestine obstruction)
Invade deep chest(myocarditis, Pericarditis, pluralities)
Bi syndrome(Brain damage)
Collapse Syn.(Shock. Ht.Kid function Failure)

(Initial stage 3 days)

(Progressive stage3-7days)

(Critic stage7-21days)

TCM Treatment of Covid-19

Initial Stage Treatment

For mild cases, home observation period.

Mild Wind-Cold Exterior and Dampness in the Interior

Signs and Symptoms: nausea, vomiting, diarrhea, abdominal pain, those often come as first symptoms especially children, fatigue, tiredness, heavy sensation, poor appetite. There will be a slight fever, cough with or without phlegm, runny nose, stuffy nose with watery discharge, sneezing, reduced taste, smell, and maybe even hearing loss.

Pale tongue body, thick, white coat

Floating, tight pulse

Treatment Principle: release exterior wind-cold, eliminate dampness, harmonize Middle Jiao

Formula: Huo Xiang Zheng Qi San

Huo Xiang Zhen Qi San (Agastache Anti-Stomach Flu Powder)

Huo Xiang	Agastache rugosa	15g
Bai Zi	Angelica dahurica	12g
Zi Su Ye	Perillae Folium	12g
Chen Pi	Citri Reticulatae Pericarpium	9g
Ban xia	Pinelliae Rhizoma	12g
Fu Ling	Poria	12g
Gan cao	Glycyrrhiza Uralensis	6g
Jie Geng	Platycodon grandiflorus (Jacq.)	9g
Hou Po	Mangnoliae Officinalis Cortex	9g

Comments

Huo Xiang Zheng Qi San is from *Peace Song Emperor Benefit People Pharmaceutical Bureau Formulas* written in the Song Dynasty. It is designed for an unseasonable evil Qi attacking the respiratory and digestive system simultaneously. It is applicable for Stomach Flu, Acute Gastritis or Acute Gastroenteritis. It was used for H1N1for a long time, and it has been adopted as a patent formula in Chinese national prevention and treatment protocol officially for COVID-19 at the initial stage.

To observe the clinical efficacy of Huo Xiang Zheng Qi San in the treatment of this new coronavirus Pneumonia, For 11cases of Chinese medicine differentiation syndrome wind cold dampness type of new coronavirus pneumonia confirmed cases had been used Huo Xiang Zheng Qi San, Results: 11 patients had pre-treatment symptom scores (8.73±5.88) and post-treatment symptom scores (0.45±0.52), and the differences before and after treatment were statistically significant (P<0.05); The main symptoms disappeared rate: fever was 100%, cough was 60%, fatigue was 100%, and white thick greasy tongue coating subsided at 64%; One of the 11 patients turned to critical condition, and the rate of critical illness was 9.09 percent, and the clinical cure rate was 100 percent. Conclusion: Huo Xiang Zheng Qi San to treat the new coronavirus pneumonia can significantly reduce the clinical symptoms of patients, prevent the transformation of mild to severe, improve the clinical cure rate, worthy of popularization and application.[1]. Yang Huanbiao etc.[J].Guang Xi Chinese Herbal Medicine. 2020. (3)1-4.

Mild Wind-Heat with Dampness

Signs and Symptoms: fever, aversion to wind, headache, runny nose with yellow discharge, thirst, sore throat, cough with or without yellow phlegm, or with nausea, vomiting, diarrhea, abdominal fullness, fatigue, tiredness, heavy sensation. Red tongue body with a thin and yellowish coating. Floating and rapid pulse. Treatment Principle: Release exterior wind-heat, restore Lungs and Wei function, eliminate dampness.

Formula:

Yin Qiao San (Golden-and-silver Honeysuckle & Forsythia powder)

written in *Detailed analysis on febrile diseases*

Add Huo Xiang, Yu Jin, Huang Qin

Jin Yin Hua	Lonicera Japonica Thunb	15g
Lian Qiao	Forsythia suspensa	15g
Niu Bang zi	Arctii Fructus	12g
Bo He	Menta piperita	12g
Jing Jie Hui	Schizonepetae Spica	9g
Dan Dou Shi	Sojae Semen Praeparatum	9g
Dan zhu Ye	Lophatherum gracile	12g
Jie Geng	Platycodon grandiflorus	12g
Lu Gen	Phragmitis Rhizoma	20g
Gan Cao	Glycyrrhiza Uralensis	6g
Huo Xiang	Agastache rugosa	15g
Yu Jin	Curcumae Radix	15g
Huang Qin	Scutellaria baicalensis Georgi	15g

Comment

Yin Qiao San is a very famous Wen Bing school formula for warmth plague at the early stage or Wei level. Not only it is acrid and cool, but also Jin Yin Hua (Lonicera Japonica), Bo He (Menta piperita), Lian Qiao (Forsythia suspensa) are aromatic which able to eliminate dampness. In his primary book, Dr. Wu, Jutong recommended to add Huo Xiang, Yu Jin aromatics to enhance the eliminating dampness effect. If there is chest and Stomach discomfort due to dampness, add Huang Qin. Yin Qiao San is applicable to H1N1, SARS, and has also been adopted as a patent formula in the national prevention and treatment protocol officially for COVID-19 at the initial stage.

To explore the mechanism of Jinhua qinggan granules (which is based on Yin Qiao San) in treating COVID-19, according to the ADME characteristics of drugs, the active ingredients and targets of Jinhua qinggan granules were screened by TCMSP platform, the component target network was constructed; The related targets of COVID-19 were retrieved based on GeneCards database; The protein-protein interaction network was constructed by String database and the key targets were screened by cytoscape software.The obtained target information was analyzed using DAVID database to analyze biological processes and pathway enrichment. Results was:263 targets of Jinhua qinggan granules and 346 COVID-19 related target genes were screened out, the mapping resulted in 49 common genes.The important gene targets were IL6, IL1β, CXCL8, CCL2, IL2, IL4, ICAM1, IL10, IFNG, IL1 A. The GO analysis results showed that the biological processes involved in the enrichment of key gene targets included cytokine activity, MAP kinase activity, chemokine activity, inflammatory response, immune response, etc.KEGG pathway analysis showed that Jinhua qinggan granules' signaling pathways for the treatment of COVID-19 included TNF signaling pathway, influenza A, HIF-1 signaling pathway, NOD-like receptor signaling pathway, Toll-like receptor signaling pathway, VEGF signaling pathway, MAPK signaling pathway, T cell receptor signaling pathway and so on.Conclusion: Jinhua qinggan granules treats COVID-19 through the multi-targets and multi-pathways mechanism of regulating immunity and reducing inflammation. [2] Study on the Network Pharmacology of Jinhua Qinggan Granules in the Treatment of COVID-19. Online Publishing Date：2020-05-12

14:38: 10.www.cnki.net

102 cases of confirmed COVID-19 has been treated with Jin Hua Qing Gan granules by Dr. Zhang Boli's team was in Wuhan city when the first outbreak happened.

Clinical studies conducted by the team at Beijing You'an Hospital found that compared with western medical groups, the number of days (7.27±3.71 days) of nucleic acid in the jinhua qinggan particle group was significantly lower than the number of days when the nucleic acid was turned negative in the control group (9.80 days) ±4.37 days), while the white blood cell renorm rate (90.2% VS 80.4%) and the lymphocyte renormalize rate (74.5% VS 64.7%) increased.[3]

Dr. Zhang Boli, a member of the Chinese Academy of Engineering said "present studies prove that the treatment using Jin Hua Qing gan granules on mild, common types of new coronavirus pneumonia shows a desirable effect. This is reflected in the shorter duration time of fever, the absorption of inflammation, the proportion of mild change to deterioration has also decreased. [4] JuXieChang Pharma Corp.Data Base. Jin Hua Qing gan granules.

Initial Stage Treatment

Damp- evil attacks the Upper Jiao (Lungs), causing Lung dysfunction and failure to disperse and descend.

Signs and Symptoms: lingering fever, chills often alternating with fever; headache, joint pain, heaviness, laziness, fatigue, reduced ability to smell, taste, even hearing loss, cough, shortness of breath, chest discomfort; nausea, vomiting, watery stool, poor appetite, no desire to drink.

Pale tongue, white thick greasy coating

Slippery, soggy, floating pulse.

Treatment Principle: Release the exterior with acrid and pungent herbs, eliminate dampness with aromatic herbs, restore the Lungs ability to disperse and descend while harmonizing the Middle Jiao.

Recommended Formulas: Hua Shi Jie Du Tang (Eliminate Dampness Detoxing Tang. (National Health Commission Protocol 8th Edition, NHCP. P.R.China. The following are the same). Mild cases use Lian Hua Clean Plague Pill (it is modified from *Jin Gui Yao Lue*).

Formula recommended by authors:

Ma Huang Jia Zhu Tang

Ma Huang	Ephedra Sinica Stapf	15g
Gui Zhi	Ramulus Cinnamomi	12g
Xing Ren	Semen Armeniacae Amarum	12g
Zhi Gan Cao	Glycyrrhiza Uralensis	6g
Bai Zhu	Atractylodes Macrocephala	12g

Modifications:

If coldness predominates replace with Ma Huang Tang

Ma Huang	Ephedra Sinica Stapf	15g
Gui Zhi	Ramulus Cinnamomi	12g
Xing Ren	Semen Armeniacae Amarum	12g
Zhi Gan Cao	Glycyrrhiza Uralensis	6g

If dampness and heat predominate: replace Ma Huang Jia Zhu Tang with Ma Xing Yi Gan Tang

Ma Huang	Ephedra Sinica Stapf	15g
Xing Ren	Semen Armeniacae Amarum	12g
Yi Yi Ren	SemenCoicis	15g
Zhi Gan Cao	Glycyrrhiza Uralensis	6g

If heat predominates: replace Ma Huang Jia Zhu Tang with Ma Xing Shi Gan Tang

Ma Huang	Ephedra Sinica Stapf	15g
Xing Ren	Semen Armeniacae Amarum	12g
Shi Gao	Gypsum Fibrosum	24g
Zhi Gan Cao	Glycyrrhiza Uralensis	6g

Comments

Ma Huang Tang is the No.1 formula in Shang Han Lun. It is mainly applicable for flu and cold-type patterns. Ma huang combined with Gui Zhi shows not only a strong antiviral, diaphoretic effect. It also acts like aspirin's antipyretic and analgesic effects. Additionally it has antihistamine, anti-congestant like effects. Ma Huang together with Xing Ren, Zhi Gan Cao has a strong antitussive effect relieving bronchial spasms. Add Bai Zhu and it becomes Ma Huang Jia Zhu Tang which is better indicated for cold-damp patterns of COVID-19. When interior dampness predominates, remove Gui Zhi from Ma Huang Tang, add Yi Yi Ren. It then becomes Ma Xing Yi Gan Tang, and when interior heat starts to predominate, add Shi Gao instead of Gui Zhi. Ma huang Tang, then becomes the famous formula Ma Xing Shi Gan Tang. Based on Ma Huang Tang, practitioners are advised to be flexible to do modifications based upon the COVID-19 case's TCM differentiation. Ma Huang leads the group of formulas and is the most common basic formula to treat on COVID-19 in China.

Lian Hua Clean Plague Pill is Ma Xing Shi Gan Tan taken from *Jin Gui Yao Lue*

(*Essential Prescriptions of the Golden Cabinet*)

The research team of the Department of Chemistry of Shantou University in Guangdong, Nanjing University of Traditional Chinese Medicine, Shanghai Pharmaceutical Research Institute of the Chinese Academy of Sciences, national key laboratory for new drug research, and the School of Life and Health Sciences of Hong Kong Chinese University (Shenzhen) published a paper online on the theoretical study of the molecular mechanism of Chinese medicine Lianhua Qing Wen against COVID-19. The researchers paired the main proteases of the virus with 21 compounds of the formula, and the results showed that the effect scores of Rutin, Hyperoside were better than those of Lopinavir. Among them, Hyperoside is the most likely inhibitor of the main protease of the new coronavirus, and it is precisely one of the main components of Lian Qiao.

The research team of Zhong Nanshan recently published a paper entitled "Lianhua Qing Wen has antiviral and anti-inflammatory effects on the new coronaviruses" in the international journal Pharmacology Research, which is the first basic research article on the effective anti-new coronavirus SARS-Cov-2 of Traditional Chinese medicine. The study found that it can significantly inhibit the replication of the new coronavirus in the cell, and the expression of viral particles in the cell decreased significantly after using this formula. A cytokine storm is an overreacting immune response in the body to external stimuli such as viruses and bacteria and becomes an important node for the development of new coronary pneumonia from mild to critical. It significantly inhibits gene over expression of genes in TNF-a, IL-6, MCP-1, and IP-10 caused by coronavirus-infected cells. This study reveals the pharmacological basis of the exact efficacy of Lianhua Qing Wen in COVID-19. The paper confirms that Lianhua Qing Wen offers an anti-corona virus activity by inhibiting viral replication and inhibiting the expression of inflammatory factors in host cells. It provides reliable evidence for the application of Lianhua Qing Wen therapy on COVID-19.

After searching seven databases and retrieving the Chinese Journal Full-text Database (CNKI), Vip Database (VIP), China Biomedicine (SinoMed), Wanfang Database and PubMed, Cochrane Central, EMBASE from October 2019 to May 2020 Literature references, included randomized controlled trials (RCTs) that tested the efficacy of the Traditional Chinese medicine Lianhuaqingwen pill in the treatment of new coronavirus pneumonia. The authors extracted data and independently assessed the quality and used Stata15.1 software to analyze the data of randomized trials.

Results showed that a total of 2 articles were identified, including 154 patients. All the participating patients were diagnosed with new coronavirus pneumonia (COVID-19). The meta-analysis results showed that the disappearance rate of the main clinical symptoms of Chinese medicine Lianhua Qingwen in the treatment of new coronavirus pneumonia was significantly higher than that of the control group [OR = 3.34, 95% CI (2.06, 5.44), P <0.001]; the disappearance rate of other clinical secondary symptoms is significantly higher than the control group [OR = 6.54, 95% CI (3.59, 11.90), P <0.001]. The duration of fever was significantly lower than that of the control group [OR = -1.04, 95% CI (-1.60, -0.49), P <0.001].

If damp turbid evil blocked in the Mo Yuanyuan (Wen Bing term refers to

interpleural-diaphragmatic space, in between exterior and interior similar to Shao Yang in Shang

Han), stubborn fever and chills happen alternatively, then add:

Da Yuan Yin from *Discussion of Epidemic Warm Disease,*

Bing Lang	Areca catechu L	15g
Cao Guo	Tsaoko Fructus	12g
Hou Po	Mangnoliae Officinalis Cortex	9g
Zhi Mu	Anemarrhenae Rhizoma	15g
Huang Qin	Scutellaria baicalensis Georgi	15g
Shao Yao	Paeonia Lactiflora Pall	12g

Eliminate Dampness Detoxing Tang, also called Q-14(Cure, 14 herbs), is the formula modified from Ma Xing Shi Gan Tang with Da Yuan Yin, which is able to restore the Lung's function of dispersing and descending strongly, calm wheezing, while eliminating damp turbidity. Of the 14 flavors of this formula, 10 drugs bind to the virus's Mpro and Spike proteins, while the remaining 4 flavors are mainly reflected in the effects on immunity, inflammation and related signaling pathways.

Initial clinical studies were carried out at the Beijing Jinyintan Hospital, East-West Lake Mobile Hospital, General Road Street Health Hospital, and efficacy was observed. 75 patients with severe cases at Jinyintan Hospital, the improvement of inflammation of the Lungs and clinical symptoms approved by CT was very obvious, and the time of nucleic acid transition and the length of hospitalization were shortened by an average of 3 days. In the General Road Street Health Hospital treatment of ordinary 124 cases, in the East and West Lake mobile Hospital randomly controlled observation of light, ordinary type 894 cases (452 cases of Chinese medicine group), confirmed the effectiveness of this formula, Liver and Kidney function tracked and tested; no adverse reactions related to Q-14 were found. In the experiment, the mouse model evaluation of the new coronavirus showed that the pulmonary tissue virus load could be reduced by 30%.

If damp heat blocks upper the Jiao/upper respiratory tract, manifested as sore throat, cough, irritability,

Use the Wen Bing formula:

Upper Jiao Disperse Blockage Tang from *Warm Diseases Analysis*

Pi Pa Ye	Eriobotrya japonica Thunb	12g
She Gan	Belamicandae Rhizome	12g
Yu Jin	Curcumae Radix	15g
Tong Cao	Akebiae Caulis	15g
Dan Dou Chi	Sojae Semen Praeparatum	9g

With alternating fever and chills always add Qing Hao, Chai Hu and Sheng Ma. With headache, body aches, joint pain, and heaviness: add Qiang Huo, Du Huo, Xi Xin, Bai Zi and Gao Ben. With frequent coughing and wheezing add Bai Bu, Zi Wan, Kuan Dong Hua, Qian Hou, Su Zi and Bai Jie Zi. With profuse phlegm and fluid add Ban Xia, Chuan Bei Mu, Gua Lou, Zhu Li, Zao Jiao, Yuan Zhi and Ze Xi.

Comments

For COVID-19, it often happens that fever and chills alternate like malaria. This is due to damp heat toxin blocking the Shao Yang Mo Yuan, which lies between the exterior and interior. Therefore, Da Yuan Yin can be added to clear Mo Yuan. If you add Qing Hao, Chai Hu and Shen Ma in the formula, it is also a good choice to clear damp heat from shao yang, harmonize shao yao, and clear toxin from shao yang.

COVID-19, which includes damp evil Qi frequently presents with headache, body ache, joint pain, therefore analgesics are needed, like Qiang Huo, Du Huo, Xi Xin, Bai Zi and Gao Ben.

Like most of the Wen Bing patterns, COVID-19 always first attacks the Lungs causing dysfunction of

the Lungs often resulting in severe cough and wheezing. Bai Bu, Zi Wan, Kuan Dong Hua are very useful, and Zi Su Zi, Bai Jie Zi are always good for controlling wheezing.

COVID-19 patients always present with copious phlegm, even profuse pink gel that obstructs the deep Lungs causing suffocation. Herbs that resolve phlegm are very helpful for the prognosis, herbs like Ban Xia, Chuan Bei Mu can dry dampness, and remove watery phlegm. Gua Lou is used for phlegm causing Lung distention with qi stagnation. Zhu Li, Zao Jiao, Yuan Zhi can dilute phlegm for sticky and difficult to expel phlegm. Ze Xi can remove watery phlegm while moving blood stasis, for cough and wheezing with cyanoderma. Zao Jiao, as a laundry nut, single use called Fishing Phlegm Pill, which can dilute phlegm and induce vomit is the best for the deep stubborn persistent phlegm case.

Progressive Stage Treatment

In this stage the pathogen has transformed to interior heat, there is Lung obstruction with heat and dampness, phlegm and fluid accumulation, this is the early stage of Lung abscess.

Signs and symptoms: severe cough, wheezing, distending chest pain; high fever, coldness, shivering, sticky sweat, yellowish smelly pus like phlegm, dry cracked skin, edema around the eyes and face, thirst, scanty yellowish urine; constipation; bloated abdomen, red tongue, yellow grey or black coating rapid pulse.

Treatment Principle: Clear heat, purge Lungs, remove phlegm, move blood stasis, and eliminate dampness.

Recommended Formulas: NHCP: Qing Fei Pai Du Tang taken from *Shang Han Lun*.

For this proposal the following formulas are recommended by the authors.

Ma Xing Shi Gan Tang modified with Wei Heng Tang

and Ting Li Da Zao Xie Fei Tang

Ma Huang	Ephedra Sinica Stapf	15g
Xing Ren	Semen Armeniacae Amarum	12g
Shi Gao	Gypsum Fibrosum	24g
Zhi Gan Cao	Glycyrrhiza Uralensis	6g
Wei Jin	Cortaderia selloana	30g
Yi Yi Ren	SemenCoicis	15g
Dong Gua Ren	Semen Benincasae	15g
Tao Ren	Semen Persicae	15g
Ting Li Zi	Draba nemorosal L	15g

Modifications

Severe Heat: add Yu Xin Cao, Chuan Xin Lian, Pu Gong Ying, Ye Ju Hua, Huang Qin, Zhi Zi, Qing Dai

Edema with scanty urine: add Fang Ji, Mu Tong, Chi Xiao Dou, Jiao Mu. Constipation with distended abdomen: add Mang Xiao, Da Huang, Hou Po, Zhi Shi. Profuse Phlegm: Jie Geng, Zao Jiao, Dan Nan Xin, Jing Ban Xia, Ze Qi. NHCP also recommends the Tan Re Qing (Phlegm heat clean) injection.

Comments

In this formula's combination, Ma Xing Shi Gan Tang is working on clearing Lung heat while dispersing and descending Lung Qi, while Wei Hen Tang focuses on nourishing body fluids, draining damp heat stagnation and clearing phlegm accumulation and blood stasis. Ting Li Zi can purge heat and fluids from Lungs, purge the bowels to calm Lung

Qi, promote urination to eliminate dampness, and lower pulmonary blood pressure.

To increase the heat clearing effect from the Lungs add Huang Qin, Zhi Zi, Pu Gong Ying, Ye Ju Hua. If there is heat fire toxin add Yu Xin Cao, Chuan Xin Lian, and Qing Dai. These are the most common combination for clearing heat fire toxin due to Lung abscess.

For high pulmonary blood pressure which often results in respiratory failure and Heart failure a diuretic protocol is a common practice. Add Fang Ji, Mu Tong, Chi Xiao Dou, Jiao Mu.

In complicated cases with Yang Ming Fu Syndrome, toxic paralytic intestinal obstruction with severe pneumonia, Lung heat can invade the Large Intestine exteriorly and interiorly, resulting in higher abdominal cavity pressure, and limited movement of the diaphragm leading to tachypnea.Add Da Chen Qi Tang to purge the bowel mechanically, and clear heat fire toxin, which often reverses the adverse condition.

Keep the airway open by resolving phlegm, for profuse Phlegm add Jie Geng, Zao Jiao, Dan Nan Xin, Jing Ban Xia, Ze Qi or use patent Tan Re Qing injection.

A large sample of multicenter retrospective cohort studies have been done with Qing Fei Pai Du Tang which is a modified Ma Xing Shi Gan Tang. It included data on 782 new coronary pneumonia in 54 hospitals in nine provinces in China. All patients were treated with Qing Fei Pai Du Tang on the basis of the use of Western medicine in accordance with the New Coronavirus Pneumonia Treatment Program (7th Edition).

Based on the time from the onset of the first clinical symptoms to the beginning of the use of QFPD

patients were divided into ≤ 1 week group (≤ 7 days), 2 weeks group (> 7 days and 14 days ≤), 3 weeks group (> 14 days and 21 days ≤) and > 3 weeks group (> 21 days) to explore the relationship between the treatment time of QFPD and clinical outcome improvement.

The results showed that the early use of QFPD in light, common patients and severe and critical patients could significantly improve the time of clinical healing, clinical recovery rate and nucleic acid time of negative days, the duration of the disease and other indicators. Compared with the treatment of QFPD after 3 weeks of symptoms for the first time, the clinical recovery time of patients treated with QFPD in early stages was significantly reduced by 2-3 times ($\leq$ 1 week group vs> 3 weeks group, 3.81, 95% CI: 2.65-5.48; 2 weeks group vs >3 weeks group: 2.63, 95% CI: 1.86-3.73; 3 weeks

group vs >3-week groups 1.92, 95% CI: 1.34-2.75); The medium time of viral nucleic acid transition was reduced from 17 days to 13 days, 12 days and 12 days respectively (Ps 0.0137); The intermediate time of the course of illness decreased from 34 days to 24 days, 21 days and 18 days (P< 0.0001); The medium length of hospitalization decreased from 18 days to 15 days, 15 days and 14 days (P< 0.0001).

The findings were published in the Lancet pre-printed platform on July 31, 2020, and once published, received widespread attention and downloads, and were eventually published in the journal Pharmacological Research (IF:5.893) under the title "Association between early treatment and Qing Fei Pai Du Decoction and favorable clinical outcomes in patients with COVID-19: A retrospective multi center cohort study."

Another study done by Prof. Li Jing included a total of 8939 patients hospitalized with new coronavirus pneumonia, of which 29% were treated with QFPD. The hospital mortality rate was 4.8% for patients who were not treated with QFPD, compared with 1.2% for patients treated with QFPD. After excluding the effects of differences in clinical characteristics and other treatments between the two groups of patients, the risk of death was only half that of patients who were treated with QFPD. And the same differences in risk of death existed between the two groups, both in patients of different ages and genders, and in various statistical analysis methods.

A study conducted at the China Huwai Hospital of National Cardiovascular Center of the Chinese Academy Medical Sciences has analyzed the medical records of nearly 10,000 cases in Hubei Province. It indicated that QFPD could halve the mortality rate of hospitalized patients with new coronavirus pneumonia. The study was published on 27 December 2020 on the internationally renowned medRxiv platform and published in the journal Phytomedicine on 31 March 2021: "Association between Qingfei Paidu Tang and mortality in hospitalized patients with COVID-19: A retrospective register study".

Critical Stage Treatment

In this stage the pathogen has transformed into fire toxins, and invades the Ying and Blood, pervades the San Jiao. There is interior obstruction and a prolapsed exterior Signs and symptoms: worsening of general condition, fever, shivering, fatigue, unclear mind, unconsciousness, delirium, harsh breathing, pain in the shoulder and chest, a feeling of suffocation, yellow face and skin, bloated and painful abdomen, constipation, scanty yellow urine or no urine hemoptysis, vomiting, hematuria, bleeding under the skin, peeling red swollen fingers on hands and feet.

Dark red tongue or black tongue, dry yellow grey black coating rapid pulse.

Cytokine storm, Systemic inflammatory response syndrome (SIRS)

For cases of fire toxins which may cause a cytokine storm due to septicemia, add clear heat and purge fire toxins formula like Huang Lian Detoxin Decoction, or traditional plague heat fire toxin strong cleaner formula Qing Wen Bai Du Yin (Clear and defeat warmth plague toxin decoction.

NHCP: RE Du Ning Injection, Yan Xi Pin Injection

Huang Lian Jie Du Tang (Huang Lian Detoxin Decoction)

Huang Qin	Scutellaria baicalensis	15g
Huang Lian	Coptis Salisb	15g
Huang Bai	Cortex Phellodendri Chinensis	15g
Zhi Zi	Gardenia Elli, nom, cons	15g

Comment

Huang Lian Jie Du Tang is a traditional formula to clear heat, purge fire, and relieve toxins. It is not only a broad spectrum antibiotics-like formula, but also a formula which can calm the cytokine storm according to pharmaceutical research.

The main active compounds of Huang lian jie du decoction were searched through TCMSP database and related literature records, and the targets of drug components were screened out.

The targets related to NCP were screened by GeneCards database. The drug-compound-target network and target protein interaction PPI network were constructed through STRING database and Cytoscape 3.6.1 software. GO enrichment and KEGG pathway annotation analysis of core targets were performed using the DAVID database.

Results were: According to the screening conditions, 60 compounds and 114 drug targets, including BCL2, PPARG, PTGS2, IFNG, etc, were obtained. The PPI core network contained 16 proteins, including MAPK1, MAPK14 and CCL2, etc. GO functional enrichment analysis obtained 43 GO items (P<0.05), KEGG pathway enrichment analysis obtained 113 pathways related to NCP (P<0.05), involving interleukin-17, hypoxia-inducible factor-1, tumor necrosis factor signaling pathway, etc.

Conclusion: The active compounds in Huang lian jie du decoction can treat the Novel Coronavirus Pneumonia by multiple targets and multiple pathways. Based on network pharmacology for mechanical study of Huang Lian Jie Du Tang treat on COVID-19. Huang, Langlang etc. Journal of Chinese medicinal materials 2020-2-29

Qing Wen Bai Du Yin is modified from Huang Lian Jie Du Tang, Bai Hu Tang and Xi Jiao Di

Huang Tang, which was successfully applied in epidemic in Qing Dynasty, supposed to be even stronger.

DIC, MIS-C (Children multiple inflammatory syndrome)

In cases where the evil has invaded the Ying and Blood Levels, DIC starts, then treatment methods are to cool the blood, move blood stasis and improve blood capillary circulation.

Recommended formulas: NHCP: Xue Bi Jin injection

For this proposal the following are recommended by authors.

Heat toxin at ying level: Qing Ying Tang

Heat toxin at blood level: Xi Jiao Di Huang Tang

Qing Ying Tang. <Detailed analysis on febrile diseases>

Xi Jiao	Rhinoceros xondaicus	2g
Shen Di Huang	Radix Rehmanniae Recens	15g
Dan sheng	Salvia miltiorrhiza Bunge	15g
Jin Yin Hua	Lonicera Japonica Thunb	15g
Liao Qiao	Forsythia suspensa	15g
Huang Lian	Coptis Salisb	12g
Dan Zhu Ye	Lophatherum gracile	12g
Xuan sheng	Scrophularia ningpoensis Hemsl	12g
Mai Meng Dong	Othiopogon japonicus	15g

Xi Jiao Di Huang Tang (Rhinoceros horn & rehmannia root cooling blood decoction)

Xi Jiao	Rhinoceros sondaicus	2g
Shen Di Huang	Radix rehmanniae Recens	15g
Chi Shao Yao	Paeonia veitchii Lynch	15g
Mu Dan Pi	Moutan Cortex	15g

Comment

It has been known that DIC (Disseminated Intravascular Coagulation) is one of the most common pathologic changes when COVID-19 is severe. It will lead to shock and multiple inner organs failure (MODS) in a short time. Qing Ying Tang and Xi Jiao Di Huang Tang are the most effective traditional formulas from the Wen Bing school.

Since both formulas above are decoctions and are hard to take, and Xi Jiao is protected animal horn, the patent Chinese Medicine formula injection Xue Bi Jing is recommended in NHCP, XBJ. It contains similar botanic herbs to cool the blood and move the blood. It has been used in the treatment of septicaemia, cytokine storm and DIC during severe pneumonia and has been proven effective.

Some doctors also suggest the use of Scopolamine injection which is an extraction from the Chinese herb Yang Jin Hua (Datura Flower). It can improve capillary blood circulation and has been applied for severe pneumonia treatment in China for many years with good efficacy.

Myocarditis

Chest binding the Heart syndrome (Myocarditis): Xiao Xian Xiong Tang

Xiao Xian Xiong Tang (Minor Chest-Draining Decoction)

Huang Lian	Coptis Salisb	15g
Ban Xia	Pinellia ternate (Thunb.) Breit	15g
Gua Lou Ren	Semen Trichosanthis	15g

Pericarditis, Pleuritis

Da Xian Xiong Tang Modified with Xiao Xian Xiong Wan

Big Chest Binding Syndrome Pericardial Effusion

Da Xian Xiong Wan (Major Chest-Draining Decoction)

Da Huang	Rheum Palmatum	15g
Mang Xiao	Natrii Sufas	12g
Ting Li Zi	Draba nemorosal L	15g
Xing Ren	Semen Armeniacae Amarum	12g

| Gan Sui | Kansui Radix | 12g |
| White Honey | Rectus mellis | 20g |

Toxic paralytic intestinal obstruction

Yang Ming Fu Shi syndrome: (Toxic paralytic intestinal obstruction): Da Chen Qi Tang Modified with Xie Bai Che Qi Tang

Da Huang	Rheum Palmatum	15g
Mang Xiao	Natrii Sufas	12g
Zhi Shi	Citrus aurantium	12g
Huo Po	Magnolia Officinalis Rehd.Et Wils	12g
Xing Ren	Semen Armeniacae Amarum	12g
Shi Gao	Gypsum Fibrosum	24g

Pleuritis with water

Xuan Ying (Pleuritis with water): Ji Jiao Li Huang Wan

Ji Jiao Li Huang Wan (Ji Jiao Li Huang Pleural Effusion Decoction) add Gan Sui

Fang Ji	Stephaniae Tetrandrae Radix	15g
Jiao Mu	Semen Zanthoxylum Bungeanum	12g
Ting Li Zi	Draba nemorosal L	5g
Da Huang	Rheum Palmatum	12g
Gan Sui	Kansui Radix	12g

Acute Kidney injury (AKI), Kidney functional failure

Dampness-Toxin pervade San Jiao, Damp heat obstructs lower Jiao, Kidney and Urinary Bladder dysfunction

Signs and Symptoms: scanty urine or no urine, lower abdominal discomforts even pain, thirsty but no desire of drinking, nausea and vomit, fever, unclear mind.

Fu Ling Pi Tang from *Detailed analysis on febrile diseases*

Add: Shi Chang Pu Yu Jin Tang modification

Fu Ling Pi	Poria	12g
Yi Yi Ren	SemenCoicis	15g
Zhu Ling	Polyporus umbellatus	12g
Da Fu Pi	Arecae Pericarpium	15g
Tong Cao	Tetrapanacis Medulla	12g
Dan Zhu Ye	Lophatherum gracile	12g
Shi Chang Pu	Acorus tatarinowii	12g
Yu Jin	Curcumae Radix	15g

Brain damage

Bi Syndrome: For Yang Bi (Brain damage): An Gong Niu Huang Wan, Zi Xue Dan, Zhi Bao Dan

(Patented formulas).

For Ying Bi: Su He Xiang Wan (Patented formula).

NHCP: Xing Nao Jing Injection

An Gong Niu HuangWan from *Detailed analysis on febrile diseases*

(Peace palace cow bezoar pill)

Niu Huang	Bos Taurus domesticus	12g
Shui Niu Jiao	Cornu Bubali	24g
She Xiang	Moschus	2g
Zhen Zhu	Margarita	9g
Zhu Sha	Cinnabaris	6g
Xiong Huang	Crocosmia Planch	6g
Huang Lian	Coptis Salisb	15g

Huang Qin	Scutellaria baicalensis Georgi	12g
Zhi Zi	Gardenia Elli, nom, cons	15g
Yu Jin	Curcumae Radix	12g
Bing Pian	Borneolum Syntheticum	9g

Zhi Bao Dan

(Top treasure pill)

Xi Jiao	Rhinoceros sondaicus	2g
Dai Mao	Eretmochelys imbricata	12g
Hu Bo	Succinum	9g
Zhu Sha	Cinnabaris	6g
Xiong Huang	Crocosmia Planch	6g
Niu Huang	Bos Taurus domesticus	12g
Long Nao	Borneolum Syntheticum	9g
She Xiang	Moschus	2g
An Xi Xiang	Styrax benzoin	9g
Golden Paper	Native gold	0.2g
Silver Paper	Native silver	0.2g

Zi Xue Dan (Blue snow powder)

Shi Gao	Gypsum Fibrosum	30g
Hua Shi	Talcum	20g
Han Shui Shi	Gypsum Rubrum	20g
Ci Shi	Magnetium Magnetite	3g
Niu Jiao	Cornu Bubali	24g
Ling Yang Jiao	Saiga tatarica Linnaeus	12g
Chen Xiang	Aquilariasinensis (Lour.) spreng	9g
Qing Mu Xiang	Radix Aristolochiae	12g
Xuan Sheng	Scrophularia ningpoensis	12g
Sheng Ma	Rhizoma Cimicifugae	12g
Zhi Gan cao	Glycyrrhiza Uralensis	6g

Ding Xiang	Syzygium aromaticum	12g
Mang Xiao	Natrii Sufas	12g
She Xiang	Moschus	2g

Su He Xiang Wan

Su He Xiang	Styrax	12g
She Xiang	Moschus	6g
Bing Pian	Borneolum	9g
Mu Xiang	RX. Aucklandiae	9g
An Xi Xiang	Benzoinum	9g
Tan Xiang	Lignum Santali Albi	12g
Ru Xiang	Olibanum	9g
Ding Xiang	Flos Caryophylli	9g
Xiang Fu	Rz.Cyperi	12g
Bi Ba	Fr.Piperis Longi	6g
Xi Jiao	Cornu Rhinoceri	6g
Zhu Sha	Cinnabaris	6g
Bai Zhu	Rz.Atractylodis Macrocephalae	12g
He Zi	Fr.Chebulae	12g

The ingredients of some formulas above are not in use because of animal protections, labour protection, or because of poisonous properties and side effects. Ingredients like Xi Jiao, Ling Yang Jiao, Zhu Sha, Xiong Huang etc. For safety, the practitioner is advised to use patent production in which producers use substitutions or omit prohibited medicinals. NHCP therefore recommended patent injection of Xingnaojing. To understand this injection, a network pharmacology of the active components of Xingnaojing and COVID-19 was established by using the method of network pharmacology.

In order to further explore the core active components and regulatory mechanism of Xingnaojing against COVID-19, the method of molecular docking was used to evaluate the binding ability of the active components in Xingnaojing with MAPK3 obtained by network pharmacology and

3CLpro that was the main protein of novel coronavirus. The results show that Xingnaojing has the characteristics of global regulation and multi-component action against COVID-19. In the active components of Xingnaojing, musk ketone, quercetin, kaempferol, naringenin and β-spisterol are the top 5 compounds that have the most binding to potential targets associated with COVID-19. The active components of Xingnaojing may bind to core targets such as MAPK3, CSF2, IL4, IL13, IL17A and TNF in the overall comprehensive regulatory process of anti-inflammatory, antiviral and immune regulation. Taking MAPK3 as an example, the prediction results of the core active components of molecular docking are basically consistent with those of network pharmacology.

Zhang Yan, Wang Qi, Li Aoqiang, Li Longjie, Wei Lin, Yan Jufen. Regulation Mechanism of Xingnaojing Injection Against COVID-19. Journal of Anhui University of Technology (Natural Science), 2021, 38(1): 49-59.

Collapse syndrome: At this stage there is shock, Heart failure, Lung failure, Liver and Kidney

failure (MODS).

Qi and Yin collapse

Sheng Mai San

| Ren Shen | Panax ginseng C.A.Mey | 12g |
| Mai Dong | Ophiopogon japonicus | 12g |

Yang Qi Collapse:

Shen Fu Tang

| Fu Zi | Aconiti Lateralis Radix Praeparata | 15g |
| Ren Shen | Panax ginseng C.A.Mey | 12g |

Heart and Kidney Yang Collapse

Si Ni Tang

Fu Zi	Aconiti Lateralis Radix Praeparata	15g
Gan Jiang	Zingiber Officinale	12g
Zhi Gan Cao	Glycyrrhiza Uralensis	6g

Recommended by NHCP: Sheng Mai Injection or Shen Fu Injection, based on the traditional formula Sheng Mai San and Shen Fu Tang.

Summary of scientific mechanical study of Chinese Medicine on COVID-19 treatment *

Disease	Pathogenesis	Chinese herbal formulas and active components	Targets and signaling pathways	Reference
Severe viral infection	Virus replication	Lianhua Qingwen formula, Wogonin (*Scutellariae Radix*), Baicalin (*Scutellariae Radix*), L-methylephedrin, L-ephedrine and D-pseudo-ephedrine (*Ephedrae Herba*), and patchouli alcohol (*Pogostemonis Herba*)	Inhibiting SARS-CoV-2, SARS-CoV, influenza A and B virus replication, inducing IFN-γ, modulating Toll-like receptors (TLRs), retinoic acid inducible gene-1 (RIG-1), adenosine monophosphate (AMP)-activated protein kinase (AMPK), phosphatidylinositol 3-kinase (PI3K)/protein kinase B (Akt), and extracellular signal-regulated kinases (ERK)/mitogen-activated protein kinase (MAPK) pathways	[23–27]
	Viral RNA synthesis	*Herba Houttuyniae*	Inhibiting SRAS-CoV RdRp	[28]
	Virus invasion	Qingfei Paidu decoction and Huoxiang Zhengqi oral liquid, patchouli alcohol, tussilagone (*Farfarae Flos*), ergosterol, asarinin (*Asari Radix et Rhizoma*), ephedrine hydrochloride (*Ephedrae Herba*), shionone (*Asteris Radix et Rhizoma*), quercetin, isorhamnetin (*Glycyrrhizae Radix et Rhizoma*), and irisolidone (*Herba Pogostemonis*)	Binding to ACE2 receptor	[29,30]
	Viral protein proteins and particle assembly	Houttuyniae Herba, Qingfei Paidu decoction and Huoxiang Zhengqi oral liquid, patchouli alcohol (*Pogostemonis Herba*), saikosaponin B (*Bupleuri Radix*), ergosterol (*Polyporus*), shionone (*Asteris Radix et Rhizoma*), 23-acetate alisol B (*Alismatis Rhizoma*), licorice glycoside E, kaempferol, (2R)-7-hydroxy-2-(4-hydroxyphenyl) chroman-4-ketone, quercetin, isorhamnetin (*Glycyrrhizae Radix et Rhizoma*), naringenin (*Citri Reticulatae Pericarpium*), robinin (*Platycodi Radix*) and irisolidone (*Herba Pogostemonis*), herbacetin (*Rhodiolae Crenulatae Radix et Rhizoma*), rhoifolin, apigenin, luteolin (*Citri Reticulatae Pericarpium*), quercetin, daidzein, and puerarin (*Puerariae Radix*)	Binding to 3CLpro and inhibiting the proteolytic activity of SARS-CoV 3CLpro	[28–31]

COVID-19 a TCM Perspective

Disease	Pathogenesis	Chinese herbal formulas and active components	Targets and signaling pathways	Reference
Inflammation and cytokine storm	Virus-infected alveolar cells release signals to recruit and activate immune cells, which secrete a variety of cytokines and chemokines and destroy the virus by releasing inflammatory mediators or phagocytosis. The excessive immune response initiates a "cytokine storm" that causes damage of lung tissue and exacerbation of pneumonia	Lianhua Qingwen capsule, *Lonicerae Japonicae Flos*, Platycodin D (*Platycodi Radix*), and *Moutan Cortex Radicis*	Suppressing pro-inflammatory cytokines production	[32–35]
		Lonicerae Japonicae Flos	Enhancing anti-inflammatory cytokines production	[33]
		Platycodin D (*Platycodi Radix*)	Suppressing apoptosis	[34]
		Platycodin D (*Platycodi Radix*) and *Moutan Cortex Radicis*	Strengthening antioxidant	[34,35]
		Platycodin D (*Platycodi Radix*) and *Moutan Cortex Radicis*	Protecting host against acute lung injury	[34,35]
		Polysaccharides of *Pinelliae Rhizoma*	Regulating IL-4 and IFN-γ	[36]
Prevention of pulmonary fluids and obstruction	Acute lung inflammation increases the permeability of lung endothelial and epithelial barriers, impairs alveolar fluids clearance mechanisms, causes edema, blocks airways, and leads to hypoxia	*Asteris Radix*, *Fritillaria cirrhosae Bulbus*, *Trichosanthis Fructus*, *Eriobotryae Japonicae Folium*, Polysaccharides of *Pinelliae Rhizoma*, and verticine	Dispelling phlegm and relieving cough, inhibiting mucus secretion in human airway epithelial cells	[36–39]
Multi-organ dysfunction	ACE2 receptor attack, immune destruction	*Astragalus* and *Angelica*, *Rheum* and its components, and triptolide	Boosting the immune system, relieving diuresis, anti-oxidation and inflammation	[40]
	Qi deficiency	*Radix Codonopsis* and *Panax ginseng*	Replenishing qi–yin deficiency, promoting organ and tissue regeneration and recovery	[21,40,41]
	Activation of the airway inflammatory pathway	Xiyanping injection (Andrographolide sulfonate)	Ameliorating airway inflammatory cell recruitment and inhibiting nuclear factor (NF)-κB and MAPK-mediated inflammatory responses	[42]
	Over-secretion of inflammatory cytokines	Xuebijing injection (*Carthamus tinctorius*, *Ligusticum wallichii*, and *Salvia miltiorrhiza*)	Suppressing inflammatory cytokine secretion	[43]
Lung fibrosis	Induction of lipogenesis	Naringenin	Inhibiting autophagy and suppressing lung inflammation and fibrosis	[44]
	Wnt signaling activation	Morusin	Alleviating mycoplasma pneumonia *via* the inhibition of Wnt/β-catenin and NF-κB signaling	[45]
	Transforming growth factor (TGF)-β and integrin activation	Yupingfeng formula (*Astragalus* and *Atractylodes macrocephala*)	Blocking fibroblast activation, collagen production, and extracellular matrix (ECM) degradation signaling pathway	[46]
	Tissue damage due to viral binding to ACE2	Tanshinone IIA	Attenuating bleomycin-induced pulmonary fibrosis *via* modulating ACE2	[47]
	p38 MAPK activation	Oxymatrine	Inhibiting phosphorylated p38 mitogen-activated protein kinase and blocking fibroblast activation and collagen production	[48]
	Activation of ECM	Honokiol	Inhibiting ECM and pro-inflammatory factors	[49,50]
	Induction of reactive oxygen Species and protein oxidation	Resveratrol and berberine	Acting as reactive oxygen species (ROS) scavenger, maintaining redox	[51–53]

*. Cite from: Engineering [J].2020.No6:10 1099-1107.

Elaine Lai-Han Leung, Hu-Dan Pan, Yu-Feng Huang, Xing-Xing Fan, Wan-Ying Wang, Fang He, Jun Cai, Hua Zhou, Liang Liu.The Scientific Foundation of Chinese Herbal Medicine against COVID-19[J]. Engineering,2020,6(10):1099-1107.

COVID-19 belongs to the warm dampness plague in Chinese medicine. The disease is in the Lungs, the pathogenesis can be summarized as dampness, heat, fire, toxin, phlegm, blood stasis. From a Western medical point of view, the genetic sequencing results of SARS-CoV-2 are highly like coronaviruses in bats and are highly consistent with most sequences in SARS-CoV. In addition, the pathological characteristics of COVID-19 are similar to those of SARS-CoV infection, and the virus enters the cell by binding the S-protein to the ACE2 receptor on the cell surface. In past studies of SARS-CoV and MERS-CoV, important drug treatment targets have been identified, such as s-protein, angiotensin conversion enzyme 2 (ACE2), TMPRSS2, coronavirus main protease (3CLpro), RNA-dependent RNA polymerase (RdRp) and papaya-like protease (PLpro) (13-16) and so on.

Many patients (80%) show mild infection or even asymptomatic, but they are highly contagious. Some patients (20%) develop rapidly into a critical/critical condition, but there are no effective drugs to alleviate the condition. Many COVID-19 patients go through five stages of progression, starting with a severe viral infection and suppression of the immune system, and cytokine storms that cause multiple organ damage and dysfunction during the transition from light to heavy. If the host has a strong immune response, the disease can also lead to complex complications such as multiple organ damage and pulmonary fibrosis

Since the similarities between SARS-CoV infection and COVID-19, the experience of Chinese medicine (CHM) in treating SARS-CoV infection 18 years ago can provide some important references to combat COVID-19, especially in the absence of special effects drugs, the use of Traditional Chinese medicine should be an important alternative therapy. Chinese medicine compound has been widely used in China in the fight against the new coronary pneumonia, its efficacy and value has also been recognized and recorded by the People's Republic of China's New

Coronary Pneumonia Treatment Program (1st-8th edition trial). As far as the treatment mechanism of Chinese herbal medicine is concerned, it has both similarities and differences with traditional Western medicine. It can play a direct antiviral role by directly interfering with the virus and the interaction between the virus and the host in virus cells, molecular targets, host receptors, signaling pathways, micro-ecological and so on.

According to the current network pharmacology research and some in vitro experiments, the mechanism of action of Chinese medicine on COVID-19 is multi-component, multi-target and multi-channel. The main mechanisms include direct antiviral action, anti-inflammatory, immunomodulation and protection of target organs. Traditional Chinese medicine itself is rich in a complex series of pharmaceutically active compounds, such as polysaccharides, flavonoids, saponins, alkaloids etc.

1. **Target SARS-CoV-2 and its host receptor ACE-2 to act as antiviral**

SARS-COV-2 is a coronavirus β membrane, single-chain, positive-chain RNA. The S protein on the surface of SARS-COV-2 induces SARS-COV-2 attachment and invasive host cells by identifying ACE2 receptors. The invading virus then controls gene replication of host cells, produces new viral RNA with RdRp, synthesizes glycoproteins through host ribosomes, is cut into nonstructural proteins and structural proteins (S proteins) by viral proteases (3CLpro and PLpro), and assembles new virus particles to release and infect other host cells. Therefore, ACE2 receptors, RdRp, Spike proteins, 3CLpro and PLpro are essential for SARS-COV-2 invasion and replication and may be potential targets for Chinese medicine for COVID-19 treatment. COVID-19 is caused by SARS-COV-2 infection of the Lungs through the respiratory tract, causing pneumonia and producing inflammatory factors, and the virus replicates and releases in the host cell, circulates in the blood, binds to ACE2 on the surface of multiple organs in the body, disrupts the balance of the RAS signaling pathway and causes damage to multiple organs throughout the body. The virus can also cause an over-immune response in the body, leading to inflammatory storms that worsen the condition, and inflammation of the Lungs produces a large amount of secretions that block the airways and exacerbate the body's hypoxia.

Traditional Chinese medicine has therapeutic effects by binding to ACE2 receptors and 3CL pro to directly inhibit the adsorption and replication of host cells by the virus. The review of Hao et al[23]. indicates that traditional Chinese medicine can be used as a supplement and alternative to primary and secondary prevention of cardiovascular disease, and its cardiovascular protection is mainly attributable to its antioxidant, anti-inflammatory and anti-cytotoxic effects [23,59]. The Heart is an organ rich in ACE2 receptors, and we speculate that the protective mechanism of Chinese medicine to the Heart is also related to this. For example, Re Du Ning injections are used in the treatment of severe COVID-19, which contains the ingredients of Dan Sheng is a typical representative cardiovascular protection in Traditional Chinese medicine. From this, we speculate that Dan Sheng in Re Du Ning injections is an active ingredient in the treatment of COVID-19 protection target organs.

In addition, even Lian Hua Qing Wen capsule has been shown to significantly and dose-dependently inhibit the replication of SARS COV-2 in the VERO E6 cells infected with SARS-COV-2 (IC50: 411.2 sg-mL-1) [32]. Yu Xin Cao have a significant inhibitory effect on 3CLpro and RdRp in SARS-COV[28]. Through network pharmacological analysis, Qing Fei Pai Du Tang and Huo Xiang Zheng Qi solution can be combined with 3CLpro and can be combined with ACE2 receptors to block the invasion and replication of SARS-COV-2 viruses [29, 30]. In addition, Hong Jin Tian, wild lacquer tree glycoside, Chen Pi, shanai phenol have also been reported to inhibit the activity of SARS-COV 3CLpro protein hydrolysis [31].

Interestingly, many active ingredients used to treat COVID-19 also have significant antiviral effects on influenza viruses. For example, jaundice effectively inhibits the replication of influenza A viruses and influenza B viruses in dog Kidney (MDCK) cells and human Lung epithelial (A549) cells by regulating the AMPK pathway. Huang Qin exhibits anti-influenza A virus (H1N1) activity both inside and outside the body and is an effective inducer of IFN-γ in the main IFN-γ preparation cells [29].

L-methyl ephedrine, L-ephedrine, and D-pseudoephedrine (ephedrine) can protect infected mice by regulating the host's TLRs and RIG-1 pathways to inhibit in vitro replication of influenza A viruses[26]. Huo Xiang has a significant inhibitory effect on the proliferation of different influenza virus A strains, and may be absorbed through cell PI3K/Akt and ERK/MAPK signaling pathway, directly inactivate the virus particles, interfere with the early stage of virus A infection, thus blocking influenza virus A infection [27].**Inhibit the pro-inflammatory cytokine and block the cytokine storm** There is growing evidence of cytokine storms in patients with severe COVID-19. IL-1B, IL-1RA, IL-6, IL-7, IL-8, IL-9, IL-10, fibroblast growth factor (FGF), granulocyte macrophage concentration stimulation factor (GM-CSF), interferon-γ, granulocyte concentration stimulation factor (G-CSF), interferon-γ Cytokine levels of γ-induced protein (IP10), immunocytochemical inducer protein 1 (MCP1), macrophage inflammatory protein 1 alpha (MIP1A), platelet-derived growth factor (PDGF), tumor necrosis factor (TNF alpha), and endothelial growth factor (VEGF) increased significantly. In critically ill or deceased patients, there was a significant increase in IL-6 levels. Clinically, through the use of a variety of anti-inflammatory treatment strategies, such as glucocorticoids, recombinant human IL-6 monoclonal antibodies, barritini (JAK inhibitors), chloroquine and hydroxychloroquine, etc.,can reduce the deterioration of fever and pneumonia, promote the absorption of pneumonia secretions, therefore, to obtain more oxygen, and improve Lung imaging performance, increase the viral negative rate. Strong evidence suggests that when treating COVID-19, the active ingredient of Traditional Chinese medicine can inhibit inflammatory cytokines, thereby alleviating cytokine storms. Li et al. studies have shown that even the level of the enchantment Lian Hua Qing Wen capsule at mRNA levels significantly reduces the level of TNF-α, IL-6, CCL-2/MCP-1 and CXCL-10/IP-10 in Huh-7 cells infected with SARS-CoV-2 infection and has concentration dependence effects. Jin Yin Hua extract can improve the binding activity of SP1 in the nucleus of cells, enhance the expression of IL-10, and reduce the expression of NF-B binding activity in acute pneumonia models in mice induced by lipid polysaccharides (LPS), thereby inhibiting the expressionof TNF-α, IL-1 beta, and IL-6[33]. Jie Geng can improve acute Lung damage induced by LPS or bolamycin by inhibiting apoptosis (reducing the expression of Caspase-3 and Bax) and inflammation (reducing TNF-α, IL-6 and NF-B), as well as by enhancing antioxidant effects (reducing the activity of myelin peroxidase (MPO) and improving the activity of superoxide dismutase). Mu Dan Pi extract can also improve acute Lung damage in LPS-induced rats by reducing the activity of IL-1 beta, MIP-2, IL-6, and MOP. Ban Xia significantly inhibit lipid polysaccharide-induced airway inflammation by regulating levels of IL-4 and IFN-h in NCI-H29 2 cells (human airway epithelial cells)and inhibiting mucus secretion.**Inhibit inflammation of the Lungs to reduce pulmonary epithelial secretion and prevent pulmonary obstruction**

Although most COVID-19 patients predominantly have fever, fatigue, and dry cough, and have a good prognosis, some severely ill patients can develop dyspnea and hypoxemia and develop rapidly into acute respiratory distress syndrome (acute respiratory syndrome, ARDS) and must use a ventilator. The pathophysiological complexity of ARDS, involving acute Lung inflammation, increases the permeability of the endothelial and epithelial barriers of the Lungs, weakens the alveoli removal mechanism, causes edema and blocks the airways, resulting in hypoxia, while the recommended Chinese medicine and its active ingredients can not only inhibit inflammation of the Lungs, slow cytokine storms, but also reduce the secretion of the epithelial Lungs, thus preventing pulmonary obstruction. For example, for more than a thousand years, chinese medicine Zi Wan, Chuan Bei Mu, Gua Lou, Pi Pa Ye and other extracts used for phlegm cough, its active ingredient has obvious effects on phlegm, cough, anti-inflammatory effect [37,39]. Traditional Chinese Medicine Can reduce the oozing of alveoli cells and vascular epithelial cells, Reduce Airway Secretion Blockage, Anti-Fibrosis. This may be the reason for improving hypoxia symptoms in patients with neo-coronavirus pneumonia, and it is also the reason for the lower probability of coVID-19 mild patients becoming too critical.

2. Protect the Lungs and multiple organs from damage

It is reported that patients with pre-existing conditions or older COVID-19 patients have a higher mortality rate because of their multiple organ failure and progression into a critical condition. Multiple organ failure is one of the leading causes of death from SARS-COV-2 infection, as SARS-COV-2 not only attacks Lung tissue, but also affects many important human organs, such as the Heart, Kidneys, testes, Liver, colon and brain. These organs express high levels of ACE2 and are therefore a key target for SARS-COV-2 attacks. Most COVID-19 patients showed typical ground glass-like change and two-sided patches in chest tomography. When a virus infects the Heart and Kidneys, it binds to ACE2 and causes cardiac arrest and Kidney failure, which is the cause of death in most patients, including those treated in the intensive care unit (ICU). Therefore, it is important to reduce viral intake, reduce symptoms and prevent disease progression at an early stage. Early applications of traditional Chinese medicine have been shown to protect vital organs and prevent the transition from mild to critical. For example, Huang Qi, Dang Gui, Da Huang can regulate the immune system by altering the proportion of Th17 cells and Th17/regulatory T-cells, relieving diuretic, antioxidant and anti-inflammatory diseases, and thus treating chronic Kidney disease [44]. Dang Sheng and Ren Shen can promote phagocytic activity and glucose metabolism pathways to treat the symptoms of Qi Deficiency in critically ill patients. Yan Xi Ping injection can improve airway inflammatory cell aggregation and inhibit the inflammatory response regulated by NF-B and MAPK. Xue Bi Ning injections inhibit the secretion of inflammatory cytokines. Although these CHMs are not directly targeted at ACE2, they can fully alleviate the patient's syndrome, increase patient comfort, and prevent further developmentof the disease.

3.   Prevention of pulmonary fibrosis

Based on experience in treating SARS-CoV infections and recent reports of COVID-19, many patients will suffer long-term Lung damage despite the low mortality rate from COVID-19. Severe patients usually develop acute viral infections, severe inflammation, alveoli epithelial cell (AEC) damage, fibroblast activation, collagen production, ECM degradation inhibition, and eventually pulmonary fibrosis, leading to Lung damage and scarring of Lung tissue. Long-term Lung damage and reduced Lung capacity will affect the patient's daily activities and quality of life after discharge from the hospital. Therefore, effective prevention of pulmonary fibrosis and rehabilitation care are also major challenges for us, and traditional Chinese medicine may help to alleviate or even reverse this pulmonary fibrosis. Therefore, Chinese medicine is also essential in the rehabilitation stage and should be widely used. In addition, although some patients have no viral load, and respiratory syndrome has been alleviated, to meet the discharge criteria, but according to Chinese medicine diagnosis, patients are usually still in a state of deficiency.

When SARS-CoV2 invades the respiratory tract and Lungs, host immune defence responses and inflammation activate the cell proliferation of epithelial cells leading to tissue regeneration. MuC5b, TGF-β, p38 MAPK, integrated prime signal conduction, Wnt signal conduction pathways in the event of infection and inflammation, most of which will be activated in the case of infection and inflammation, and will also cause the induction of reactive oxygen (ROS). It will open up the cell cycle regulation gene, which leads to the proliferation of pulmonary fibroblasts. ROS also induces protein oxidation, which is associated with inflammatory reactions associated with cell damage, eventually leading to pulmonary fibrosis and blockages. In addition, cell aging, mitochondrial dysfunction, and protein stabilization disorders are also causes of pulmonary fibrosis. Drugs can prevent pulmonary fibrosis by suppressing these factors, especially in the early stages of the disease.

Previous studies have shown that some medicinal plants, traditional Chinese medicines, and their active ingredients can reduce pulmonary fibrosis caused by a variety of pneumonias, including SARS-CoV. Therefore, we recommend the early use of Traditional Chinese medicine to treat COVID-19 to block these pathways and pulmonary fibrosis. Jade screen is an herbal formula consisting of Huang Qi, Bai Zhu, Fang Feng, which inhibits the cell proliferation stimulation signal of TGF-β, hindering the activation of fibroblasts and the production of collagen [49]. In addition, it has been reported that Chen Pi inhibits autophagy by reducing ROS, thereby suppressing pneumonia and fibrosis [65],and Sang Bai Pi reduces mycoplasma pneumonia by inhibiting Wnt/β serial proteins and NF-B signals [75]. Dan Shen inhibits the virus binding to regulate ACE2, it weakens bleomycin-induced pulmonary fibrosis[50] ,Ku Shen can inhibit phosphorylation of p38 fissile protein kinase cell proliferation signal[51] .

Even after the patient is discharged from the hospital, there may still be a Qi and Yin deficiency, depression or other discomfort requiring further treatment. Ren Shen and Huang Qi are commonly used in clinical practice and have shown remarkable results in preventing experimental pulmonary fibrosis [69,70]. It has been reported that Hou Po can also inhibit proinflammatory factors and reduce pulmonary fibrosis [52,53]. In addition, some compounds extracted from Chinese medicine can be used as ROS scavengers, such as resveratrol, berberine, etc. they may target redox imbalances to reduce inflammation and fibrosis in the Lungs.[80,82]

In summary, the pathogenesis of COVID-19 was identified with the identification of therapeutic targets and potential treatment strategies, and antiviral drugs, IL-6 inhibitors, IFN-γ, immunosuppressants, oxygen therapy and support therapies were recommended for the treatment of COVID-19 patients, at all different stages in COVID-19 patients, TCM can achieve therapeutic results through multidimensional pathways and targets.

Reference:

[21] Jiang WY. Therapeutic wisdom in traditional Chinese medicine: a perspective from modern science. Trends Pharmacol Sci 2005;26(11):558–63.

[22] Yuan R, Lin Y. Traditional Chinese medicine: an approach to scientific proof and clinical validation. Pharmacol Ther 2000;86(2):191–8.

[23] Hao PP, Jiang F, Chen YG, Yang J, Zhang K, Zhang MX, et al. Traditional Chinese medication for cardiovascular disease. Nat Rev Cardiol 2015;12(2):115–22.

[24] Seong RK, Kim JA, Shin OS. Wogonin, a flavonoid isolated from Scutellaria baicalensis, has antiviral activities against influenza infection via modulation of AMPK pathways. Acta Virol 2018;62(1):78–85.

[25] Chu M, Xu L, Zhang M, Chu Z, Wang Y. Role of Baicalin in anti-influenza virus A as a potent inducer of IFN-c. BioMed Res Int 2015;2015:263630.

[26] Wei W, Du H, Shao C, Zhou H, Lu Y, Yu L, et al. Screening of antiviral components of Ma Huang Tang and investigation on the ephedra alkaloids efficacy on influenza virus type A. Front Pharmacol 2019;10:961.

[27] Yu Y, Zhang Y, Wang S, Liu W, Hao C, Wang W. Inhibition effects of patchouli alcohol against influenza a virus through targeting cellular PI3K/Akt and ERK/ MAPK signaling pathways. Virol J 2019;16(1):163.

[28] Lau KM, Lee KM, Koon CM, Cheung CSF, Lau CP, Ho HM, et al. Immunomodulatory and anti-SARS activities of Houttuynia cordata. J Ethnopharmacol 2008;118(1):79–85.

[29] Zhang D, Zhang B, Lv JT, Sa RN, Zhang XM, Lin ZJ. The clinical benefits of Chinese patent medicines against COVID-19 based on current evidence. Pharmacol Res 2020;157:104882.

[30] Deng Y, Liu B, He Z, Liu T, Zheng R, Yang A, et al. Study on active compounds from Huoxiang Zhengqi Oral Liquid for prevention of coronavirus disease 2019 (COVID-19) based on network pharmacology and molecular docking. Chin Tradit Herbal Drugs 2020;51(5):1113–22.

[31] Jo S, Kim S, Shin DH, Kim MS. Inhibition of SARS-CoV 3CL protease by flavonoids. J Enzyme Inhib Med Chem 2020;35(1):145–51.

[32] Li R, Hou Y, Huang J, Pan W, Ma Q, Shi Y, et al. Lianhuaqingwen exerts anti-viral and anti-inflammatory activity against novel coronavirus (SARS-CoV-2). Pharmacol Res 2020;156:104761.

[33] Kao ST, Liu CJ, Yeh CC. Protective and immunomodulatory effect of flos Lonicerae japonicae by augmenting IL-10 expression in a murine model of acute Lung inflammation. J Ethnopharmacol 2015;168:108–15.

[34] Tao W, Su Q, Wang H, Guo S, Chen Y, Duan J, et al. Platycodin D attenuates acute Lung injury by suppressing apoptosis and inflammation in vivo and in vitro. Int Immunopharmacol 2015;27(1):138–47.

[35] Fu PK, Yang CY, Tsai TH, Hsieh CL. Moutan cortex radicis improves lipopolysaccharide-induced acute Lung injury in rats through anti inflammation. Phytomedicine 2012;19(13):1206–15.

[36] Hu M, Liu Y, Wang L, Wang J, Li L, Wu C. Purification, characterization of two polysaccharides from Pinelliae Rhizoma Praeparatum cum Alumine and their anti-inflammatory effects on mucus secretion of airway epithelium. Int J Mol Sci 2019;20(14):3553.

[37] Xu Y, Ming TW, Gaun TKW, Wang S, Ye B. A comparative assessment of acute oral toxicity and traditional pharmacological activities between extracts of Fritillaria cirrhosae Bulbus and Fritillaria pallidiflora Bulbus. J Ethnopharmacol 2019;238:111853.

[38] Yu P, Cheng S, Xiang J, Yu B, Zhang M, Zhang C, et al. Expectorant, antitussive, anti-inflammatory activities and compositional analysis of Aster tataricus. J Ethnopharmacol 2015;164:328–33.

[39] Yu X, Tang L, Wu H, Zhang X, Luo H, Guo R, et al. Trichosanthis Fructus: botany, traditional uses, phytochemistry and pharmacology. J Ethnopharmacol 2018;224:177–94.

[40] Wang D, Hu B, Hu C, Zhu F, Liu X, Zhang J, et al. Clinical characteristics of 138 hospitalized patients with 2019 novel coronavirus-infected pneumonia in Wuhan, China. JAMA 2020;323(11):1061–9.

[41] Szodoray P, Nakken B, Barath S, Csipo I, Nagy G, El-Hage F, et al. Altered Th17 cells and Th17/regulatory T-cell ratios indicate the subsequent conversion from undifferentiated connective tissue disease to definitive systemic autoimmune disorders. Hum Immunol 2013;74(12):1510–8.

[42] Peng S, Hang N, Liu W, Guo W, Jiang C, Yang X, et al. Andrographolide sulfonate ameliorates lipopolysaccharide-induced acute Lung injury in mice by downregulating MAPK and NF-jB pathways. Acta Pharm Sin B 2016;6(3):205–11.

[43] Song Y, Yao C, Yao Y, Han H, Zhao X, Yu K, et al. XueBiJing injection versus placebo for critically III patients with severe community-acquired pneumonia: a randomized controlled trial. Crit Care Med 2019;47(9): e735–43.

[44] Chen Y, Nie Y, Luo Y, Lin F, Zheng Y, Cheng G, et al. Protective effects of naringin against paraquat-induced acute Lung injury and pulmonary fibrosis in mice. Food Chem Toxicol 2013;58:133–40.

[45] Cui W, Li L, Li D, Mo X, Zhou W, Zhang Z, et al. Total glycosides of Yupingfeng protects against bleomycin-induced pulmonary fibrosis in rats associated with reduced high mobility group box 1 activation and epithelial-mesenchymal transition. Inflamm Res 2015;64(12):953–61.

[46] Xia H, Diebold D, Nho R, Perlman D, Kleidon J, Kahm J, et al. Pathological integrin signaling enhances proliferation of primary Lung fibroblasts from patients with idiopathic pulmonary fibrosis. J Exp Med 2008;205(7):1659–72.

[47] Stewart AG, Thomas B, Koff J. TGF-b: master regulator of inflammation and fibrosis. Respirology 2018;23(12):1096–7.

[48] Somogyi V, Chaudhuri N, Torrisi SE, Kahn N, Müller V, Kreuter M. The therapy of idiopathic pulmonary fibrosis: what is next? Eur Respir Rev 2019;28 (153):190021.

[49] Li L, Li D, Xu L, Zhao P, Deng Z, Mo X, et al. Total extract of Yupingfeng attenuates bleomycin-induced pulmonary fibrosis in rats. Phytomedicine 2015;22(1):111–9.

[50] Wu H, Li Y, Wang Y, Xu D, Li C, Liu M, et al. Tanshinone IIA attenuates bleomycin-induced pulmonary fibrosis via modulating angiotensin converting enzyme 2/angiotensin-(1–7) axis in rats. Int J Med Sci 2014;11 (6):578–86.

[51] Dong J, Ma Q. Osteopontin enhances multi-walled carbon nanotube-triggered Lung fibrosis by promoting TGF-b1 activation and myofibroblast differentiation. Part Fibre Toxicol 2017;14(1):18.

[52] Chiang CK, Sheu ML, Lin YW, Wu CT, Yang CC, Chen MW, et al. Honokiol ameliorates renal fibrosis by inhibiting extracellular matrix and proinflammatory factors in vivo and in vitro. Br J Pharmacol 2011;163 (3):586–97.

[53] Weng TI, Wu HY, Kuo CW, Liu SH. Honokiol rescues sepsis-associated acute Lung injury and lethality via the inhibition of oxidative stress and inflammation. Intensive Care Med 2011;37(3):533–41.

[54] Huang YF, Bai C, He F, Xie Y, Zhou H. Review on the potential action mechanisms of Chinese medicines in treating coronavirus disease 2019 (COVID-19). Pharmacol Res 2020;158:104939.

[55] Wang WY, Xie Y, Zhou H, Liu L. Contribution of traditional Chinese medicine to the treatment of COVID-19. Phytomedicine 2020. In the press.

[56] Kiemer L, Lund O, Brunak S, Blom N. Coronavirus 3CLpro proteinase cleavage sites: possible relevance to SARS virus pathology. BMC Bioinf 2004;5(1):72.

[57] Thiel V, Ivanov KA, Putics Á, Hertzig T, Schelle B, Bayer S, et al. Mechanisms and enzymes involved in SARS coronavirus genome expression. J Gen Virol 2003;84(9):2305–15.

[58] Li G, De Clercq E. Therapeutic options for the 2019 novel coronavirus (2019- nCoV). Nat Rev Drug Discov 2020;19(3):149–50.

[59] Hao P, Jiang F, Cheng J, Ma L, Zhang Y, Zhao Y. Traditional Chinese medicine for cardiovascular disease: evidence and potential mechanisms. J Am Coll Cardiol 2017;69(24):2952–66.

[60] Wan S, Yi Q, Fan S, Lv J, Zhang X, Guo L, et al. Characteristics of lymphocyte subsets and cytokines in peripheral blood of 123 hospitalized patients with 2019 novel coronavirus pneumonia (NCP). 2020. medRxiv:2020.02.10.20021832.

[61] Huang C, Wang Y, Li X, Ren L, Zhao J, Hu Y, et al. Clinical features of patients infected with 2019 novel coronavirus in Wuhan, China. Lancet 2020;395 (10223):497–506.

[62] Ruan Q, Yang K, Wang W, Jiang L, Song J. Clinical predictors of mortality due to COVID-19 based on an analysis of data of 150 patients from Wuhan, China. Intensive Care Med 2020;46(5):846–8.

[63] Chen N, Zhou M, Dong X, Qu J, Gong F, Han Y, et al. Epidemiological and clinical characteristics of 99 cases of 2019 novel coronavirus pneumonia in Wuhan, China: a descriptive study. Lancet 2020;395(10223):507–13.

[64] Wu C, Chen X, Cai Y, Xia J, Zhou X, Xu S, et al. Risk factors associated with acute respiratory distress syndrome and death in patients with coronavirus disease 2019 pneumonia in Wuhan, China. JAMA Intern Med 2020;180 (7):1–11.

[65] Zhang W, Zhao Y, Zhang F, Wang Q, Li T, Liu Z, et al. The use of antiinflammatory drugs in the treatment of people with severe coronavirus disease 2019 (COVID-19): the perspectives of clinical immunologists from China. Clin Immunol 2020;214:108393.

[66] Ware LB. Pathophysiology of acute respiratory distress syndrome. In: Webb A, Angus D, Finfer S, Gattinoni L, Singer M, editors. Oxford textbook of critical care. Oxford: Oxford University Press; 2016. p. 497–500.

[67] Chai X, Hu L, Zhang Y, Han W, Lu Z, Ke A, et al. Specific ACE2 expression in cholangiocytes may cause Liver damage after 2019-nCoV infection. 2020. bioRxiv:2020.02.03.931766.

[68] Xu YH, Dong JH, An WM, Lv XY, Yin XP, Zhang JZ, et al. Clinical and computed tomographic imaging features of novel coronavirus pneumonia caused by SARS-CoV-2. J Infect 2020;80(4):394–400.

[69] Yuen MF, Tam S, Fung J, Wong DKH, Wong BCY, Lai CL. Traditional Chinese medicine causing hepatotoxicity in patients with chronic hepatitis B infection: a 1-year prospective study. Aliment Pharmacol Ther 2006;24(8):1179–86.

[70] Kam PC, Liew S. Traditional Chinese herbal medicine and anaesthesia. Anaesthesia 2002;57(11):1083–9.

[71] McLean-Tooke A, Moore I, Lake F. Idiopathic and immune-related pulmonary fibrosis: diagnostic and therapeutic challenges. Clin Transl Immunol 2019;8 (11): e1086.

[72] Otoupalova E, Smith S, Cheng G, Thannickal VJ. Oxidative stress in pulmonary fibrosis. Compr Physiol 2020;10(2):509–47.

[73] Divya T, Dineshbabu V, Soumyakrishnan S, Sureshkumar A, Sudhandiran G. Celastrol enhances Nrf2 mediated antioxidant enzymes and exhibits anti-fibrotic effect through regulation of collagen production against bleomycin-induced pulmonary fibrosis. Chem Biol Interact 2016;246:52–62.

[74] Nakahira K, Pabon Porras MA, Choi AM. Autophagy in pulmonary diseases. Am J Respir Crit Care Med 2016;194(10):1196–207.

[75] Chen C, Wang J, Chen J, Zhou L, Wang H, Chen J, et al. Morusin alleviates mycoplasma pneumonia via the inhibition of Wnt/b-catenin and NF-jB signaling. Biosci Rep 2019;39(6): BRS20190190.

[76] Williamson JD, Sadofsky LR, Hart SP. The pathogenesis of bleomycin-induced Lung injury in animals and its applicability to human idiopathic pulmonary fibrosis. Exp Lung Res 2015;41(2):57–73.

[77] Kitamura H, Cambier S, Somanath S, Barker T, Minagawa S, Markovics J, et al. Mouse and human Lung fibroblasts regulate dendritic cell trafficking, airway inflammation, and fibrosis through integrin avb8-mediated activation of TGFb. J Clin Invest 2011;121(7):2863–75.

[78] Weng T, Ko J, Masamha CP, Xia Z, Xiang Y, Chen NY, et al. Cleavage factor 25 deregulation contributes to pulmonary fibrosis through alternative polyadenylation. J Clin Invest 2019;129(5):1984–99.

[79] Borok Z. Role for a3 integrin in EMT and pulmonary fibrosis. J Clin Invest 2009;119(1):7–10.

[80] Sato N, Takasaka N, Yoshida M, Tsubouchi K, Minagawa S, Araya J, et al. Metformin attenuates Lung fibrosis development via NOX4 suppression. Respir Res 2016;17(1):107.

[81] Kheirollahi V, Wasnick RM, Biasin V, Vazquez-Armendariz AI, Chu X, Moiseenko A, et al. Metformin induces lipogenic differentiation in myofibroblasts to reverse Lung fibrosis. Nat Commun 2019;10(1):2987.

[82] Rangarajan S, Bone NB, Zmijewska AA, Jiang S, Park DW, Bernard K, et al. Metformin reverses established Lung fibrosis in a bleomycin model. Nat Med 2018;24(8):1121–7.

Chapter Four

TCM Treatment of Post Covid-19

TCM approach in treating long-term symptoms of Covid-19

There is no specific test to diagnose patients with long-term symptoms of Covid-19. This group is mixed in with those who experienced both mild and severe cases. People from all demographics can have long-term effects. This includes patients across all age groups as well as those with or without pre-existing conditions. Ten percent of Covid-19 patients become long haulers with symptoms lasting 2-3 months after initial infection. If symptoms last longer than 28 days, they can be considered long-term patients. It is not completely clear at this time whether or not long haulers are still contagious or not. Long lasting symptoms may themselves create a health crisis.

Some key points on Covid-19 immune response:

- Covid-19 antigen will reach the peak 15 days from initial infection, it is no longer detectable after four weeks.
- The patient will either die from the disease in four weeks or covid 19 antigen will be eliminated by antibodies IgM, IgG or by antivirus medicine.
- Covid-19 virus may only have four weeks life, and the patient is considered not contagious after three weeks of quarantine.
- It may be safer to work on long lasting covid 19 patients.

- After Covid-19 infection the patient's immune system produces antibodies IgM from day 7 to day 21, it will reach the peak on day 15, and will be undetectable after three weeks.
- IgG antibodies (long – term antibodies) will be produced on day 14, on the other hand, the immune system needs two weeks to produce IgG, it will reach the peak in the 4th week and last more than three months or a year.
- IgM will be detectable after the first week, no longer detectable after three weeks.
- IgG will be detectable after two weeks and stay positive for months to a year, it is usually used as a marker of immunity.

The theory what causes chronic Covid-19 symptoms:

- Remnants of viral material possibly remain in the body at undetectable levels.
- Patient's immune systems continue to overreact even though the infection has passed, though there seems to be no consistent reason for this to happen.

Common Long Hauler Symptoms

Patients experiencing long lasting symptoms may include fatigue, loss of taste and smell, shortness of breath, difficulty sleeping, anxiety, brain fog, poor memory, depression, body aches, coughing, headache, Stomach discomfort, nausea, insomnia and tinnitus.

Long-term Covid-19 symptoms pattern A

Manifestations: fatigue, insomnia, poor memory, brain fog, the pulse is weak, thin and rapid, the tongue is pale and swollen

Treatment Strategy: supplement Qi and blood, clear infection

Formula: Ba Zhen Tang, Tian Wang Bu Xin Dan, Qi Xue Da Bu Wan, Shen Qi Da Bu Wan

Acupuncture points: Ren4, 14, Du3, 14, 20, St36, Sp10, Li4, Ht7, AnMian

Ear Magnets- shen men, Heart, Kidney. Stimulate the magnets for 20 seconds/hour

Jade Turtle Breathing- 5 second inhale, 5 second exhale, 5 second breath hold

Supplements: CoQ10, Vitamins B, A, D

Long-term Covid-19 symptoms pattern B

Manifestations: anxiety, depression, fatigue, poor cognition, insomnia, thin, rapid and wiry pulse, pale tongue with red edges and a white coating

Treatment Strategy: soothe and regulate Qi, nourish yin, clear heat, clear infection

Formula: Yi Guan Jian, Xiao Yao San, Si Ni San, Suan Zao Ren Wan. An antiviral combination contains Jin Yin Hua, Lian Qiao, Chai Hu, Da Qing Ye, Huang Qin, Jie Geng, Chuan Xin Lian, Ban Lan Gen, Qiang Huo.

Acupuncture points: Lv2,3, P6, 7, Ki3, Gb20, Ren17, Sp9, Li11, 4

Ear Magnets: Heart, Kidney, Liver

Long-term Covid-19 symptoms pattern C

Manifestations: loss of taste and smell, headache, Stomach discomfort, nausea, deep and thin pulse, pale, swollen tongue with thin and white coating

Treatment Strategy: nourish and smooth Qi, move stagnation, clear infection

Formula: Ren Shen Bai Du Wan, Cang Er Zi San

Acupuncture points: Du4, 14, 20, Ren 4, 14, 20, Li4, 20, St 3, 6, 7, 43, 36, Lv3

Ear Magnets: shen men, Stomach, Lung, magnets on P6 and SJ5 for five days.

Supplements: CoQ10, Vitamins A, B, D

Long-Lasting Covid-19 symptoms pattern D

Manifestations: shortness of breath, fatigue, cough, weak, thin and rapid pulse, pale and purple tongue with thin and white coating

Treatment Strategy: nourish and regulate Qi, dispel dampness

Formula: Ke Chuan Wan, San Zi Yang Qin Wan, Su Zi Jiang Qi Wan, Qing Qi Hua Tan Tang

Acupuncture points: Ren4, 14, 17, 20, 22, Ki 3, 27, Li4, 20, Bl11, 13, 15, 23, Du 2, 4, 14, 20

Ear Magnets: shen men, Kidney, Lung. Stimulate every hour

Press tacks: Du14, Ding Chuan, retain for 3 days

Plum Blossom hammer: Du14, Bl11, 13, 15, 23

Cupping: DU3, 14, Ren 4, 19, BL11, 13, 15

Long-Lasting Covid-19 symptoms Pattern E

Manifestations: severe nausea, Stomachache, abdominal cramping and bloating, hunger without desire to eat, no appetite, constipation, low energy, insomnia, thin and rapid pulse, pale tongue with light yellow coating

Formula: Su Zi Huang Lian Tang, Si Ni San

Acupuncture points: Ren 4, 6, 14, 20, Du 3, 14, 23, SJ5, P6, St43, 36, 43, Lv3

Ear Magnets: Stomach, shen men, Liver. Place magnets on SJ5 and P6 for 5 days, stimulate hourly

Long-Lasting Covid-19 symptoms pattern F

Manifestations: vertigo, dizziness, shock, fear, shortness of breath, crying, thin, rapin and tight pulse, tongue with red edges with thin and yellow coat

Treatment Strategy: clear heat, drain dampness, clear infection

Formula: Ban Xia Bai Zhu Tian Ma Tang, Ban Xia Xie Xin Wan

Acupuncture points: Li4, 11, St36, 40, 44, Lv3, Ren4,14, Yi Feng, Jian Er

Ear Magnets: Liver, shen men

Long-Lasting Covid-19 symptoms pattern G

Manifestations: headache in whole head, neck pain, back pain, all over body pain, fever, shortness of breath, extreme fatigue, thin, rapid and wiry pulse, tongue is pale and purple.

Treatment strategy: regulate and nourish Qi, remove stagnation

Formula: Ren Shen Bai Du San, Tian Ma Wan, Pu Ji Xiao Du Yin, Juan Bi Tang

Acupuncture points. St8, 36, Du 3, 14, 20, 23, BL11, 13, 15, 23, Lv3, 8, Ren 4, 14, GB20 Da Cha Xue

Self-care: patient should use a heating pad on all painful areas, perform scalp massage with White Flower Oil.

Differentiation and treatment plan:

Qi stagnation and deficiency

Regulate and nourish Qi.

Points and Herbs

1. S8, 36, 43. GV3,14,20,23. B11, 13,15,23. Lr3,8. CV4,14. GB20. Da Cha Xue
2. White Flower Oil few drops put on temples, forehead during acupuncture treatment.
3. Self-Healing Scalp Massage with White Flower Oil
4. Teaching patients how to do it and let patients do it 4-5 times a day.
5. Ren Seng Bai Du San + Tian Ma Wan
6. Pu Ji Xiao Du Yin Juan Bi Tang Wan.
7. Doctor order: put heating pad on neck back or body pain spots 30 minutes twice a day.

Additional thoughts:

- Long haulers symptoms are quite improvable.
- It seems necessary to use anti-virus herbs in early treatment to clear residual virus
- Most long haulers are qi, blood, yin, yang deficient, or some residual heat and stagnation.
- Nourishing qi, clearing heat, and regulating qi always work well.
- Long lasting symptoms respond effectively well to TCM therapies.

Chronic Fatigue Post Covid-19

Over half of the people who recover from COVID-19 report fatigue 10 weeks later, regardless of the seriousness of their initial infection. It is a long-term illness that affects several body systems. It is especially important for people with increased risk of severe illness from COVID-19 to protect themselves. In addition it is very important to treat the disease quickly in order to avoid post-Covid 19 fatigue. TCM has been used to treat post-Covid 19 fatigue and has offered successful results for patients around the world.

In TCM, the post-Covid 19 fatigue might be referred to Lassitude (倦怠 Juan Dai), deficient syndrome (虚损Xu Sun). Dr Xue Shengbai in his book, *the Damp Warm Febrile Disease* says: The illness just occurs during the summer, as long as there are chills, yellow face, no thirst, fatigue, weakness in the extremities, deep and weak pulse, painful abdomen and loose stool. This is due to dampness accumulating in the Yang of Taiyin. The Suo Pi Yin, Da Sun San and Lai Fu Dan are useful.

Etiology, Pathogenesis and Therapy

Dampness lingers during most of the stages of Covid 19, it consumes Spleen yang or damages yin of the Lung, Stomach, Heart, Liver and Kidney. The location of the disease mechanism focuses on the Spleen and affects other Zang Fu organs. There is deficiency during the post-Covid 19 infection. These deficiencies include Qi, Blood, Yin and Yang deficiency of all Zang Fu organs. There may also be excess, such as Qi stagnation and damp phlegm accumulation.

Liver and Kidney Yin deficiency

In older patients with the Yin deficient constitutions, post Covid-19 pathogens typically turn to heat leading to damage of Liver and Kidney Yin. The Yin deficiency of Liver and Kidney leads to failure in nourishing the bones and tendons. This manifests as low back and knee pain, hot flashes and night sweats.

Manifestations: fatigue, low back and knee pain, hot flashes, night sweats, thirst, constipation, light or irregular period, premature ejaculation, tinnitus, dizziness, red tongue with scanty or peeled coating, deep, weak, and rapid pulse.

Treatment Strategy: Nourish the Yin of the Liver and Kidney.

Formula: Liu Wei Di Huang Wan.

Qi Ju Di Huang Wan can be used if the patient has severe tinnitus and dizziness. Zhi Bai Di Huang Wan can be used if the patient has more hot flashes, night sweats, and a burning sensation with urination.

Acupuncture points: UB18, UB23, Ki3, Liv3, GB20.

Lung and Heart Qi, Yin deficiency

The damp toxin of Covid-19 damages the Qi and Yin of the Heart. Lung Qi fails to take charge of Qi manifesting as fatigue, shortness of breath and a weak voice. The Lung and Heart Yin is injured and fails to nourish yin, manifesting as a dry cough, dry mouth, palpitations, and mental depression.

Manifestations: fatigue, shortness of breath, weak voice, dry cough, dry mouth, palpitations, mental depression, small and pale tongue without coating, deep weak and rapid pulse.

Treatment Strategy: Tonify the Qi and nourish the Yin of the Lung and Heart.

Formula: Sheng Mai San modified.

If there is anxiety, palpitations and insomnia, add Dan Shen and Huang Qi. If there is a chronic cough, Bu Fei Tang can be added.

Acupuncture points: Lu1, PC6, Ki6, St36, Ren17.

Heart and Spleen deficiency

The Spleen is affected by dampness during Damp, Warm febrile diseases. It can also be injured by the overuse of cold and bitter herbs. When these occur the Spleen fails to generate the Qi and Blood and to nourish the Heart, therefore the patient has the manifestations of both Heart and Spleen deficiency.

Manifestations: fatigue, lassitude, insomnia, palpitations, poor appetite, pale complexion, pale lips and tongue and deep weak pulse.

Treatment Strategy: Supplement the Qi and blood of Heart and Spleen.

Formula: Gui Pi Tang.

If there is severe insomnia and dream disturbed sleep, add Suan Zao Ren and Ye Jiao Teng.

Acupuncture Points: Ren14, Ren12, Sp6, Ht7, Anmian.

Middle Qi deficiency:

Dampness lingering inside, delay in treatment or incorrect therapy results in Spleen Qi deficiency. The Spleen then fails to generate Qi and to nourish the muscles manifesting as lassitude and weakness of the muscles. When the clear Qi fails to ascend and nourish the brain, the patient will have fatigue, dizziness, and loose stool.

Manifestations: fatigue, lassitude, dizziness, poor appetite, loose stool, pale tongue with thin white coating, deep and weak pulse.

Treatment Strategy: Supplement the middle Qi.

Formula: Liu Jun Zi Tang.

Liu Jun Zi Tang is mostly used for fatigue, lassitude, poor appetite, and loose stool due to the Qi deficiency of Spleen and Stomach. It also can be used for Lung and Spleen Qi deficiency with dampness and phlegm manifesting as fatigue, chronic cough with phlegm and pale tongue with white greasy coating. Bu Zhong Yi Qi Tang is used for fatigue and dizziness due to prolapsed middle Qi.

Acupuncture Points: Du20, Ren12, St36, Sp6, SP4.

Spleen Yang deficiency with dampness:

The damp aspect of Covid-19 injures Spleen Yang, which especially occurs in patients with underlying Yang deficiency. Spleen, even Kidney Yang deficiency results in overflow of water and dampness with lassitude, fatigue, and puffy face.

Manifestations: Fatigue, heavy sensation of the body, puffy face, diarrhea, and edema of limbs, bloating abdomen, pale and swollen tongue with white and greasy coating, deep and weak pulse.

Treatment Strategy: Warm the Spleen Yang and eliminate dampness.

Formula: Fu Zi Li Zhong Tang.

For significant edema due to Yang deficiency of Spleen and Kidney, add Zhen Wu Tang.

Acupuncture points: Ren12, Ren6 (Moxa), St36, Du4(Moxa), SJ5, Sp9.

Liver Qi stagnation with Spleen Qi deficiency:

A global pandemic is going to be met with severe stress that will affect all kinds of people no matter what their background or lifestyle. Chronic stress results in Liver Qi stagnation that leads to excessive Liver Qi attacking the Spleen.

Manifestations: fatigue, rib-side, abdominal bloating, poor appetite, loose stool, pale tongue with thin white coating, wiry pulse at left, deep and weak pulse at right.

Treatment Strategy: soothe Liver Qi and supplement Spleen Qi.

Formula: Xiao Yao San.

For significant Liver Qi stagnation, add Xiang Fu, Zhi Shi. For severe fatigue with Qi deficiency, add Huang Qi, and Ren Shen. For depression and poor sleep, add He Huan Pi and Ye Jiao Teng.

Acupuncture Points: Yintang, Liv13, LI4, Liv3, Ren12.

Additional therapies

Cupping: Moving Cupping along Huatuojiaji and the back Shu of UB channel

Guasha: Push Guasha along the Du, Ren, and UB channel.

Xie Wei Tie Fu: use Ren Shen, Shan Zhu Yu, Fu Zi and Rou Gui (1:1:1:1), 0.5g put on each point at five back Shu, Du4, and Ren3. It is used for fatigue due to deficiency of the five Zang Organs.

PTSD Post Covid-19

COVID-19 has quickly become a global health emergency resulting in not only physical health concerns but also psychological concerns as people are exposed to unexpected deaths or threats of death. For example, healthcare workers who have close contact with COVID patients are not only exposed to the virus on a regular basis, but they may also be witnessing increased illnesses, deaths, and supply shortages. In addition, patients admitted to the hospital with COVID-19 experience social isolation, physical discomfort, and fear for survival. These exposures increase the risk of developing Post-traumatic stress disorder (PTSD). In addition, the risk may further be enhanced during the subsequent weeks when these individuals may lack immediate social support due to the need to self-quarantine.

PTSD might be referred to as an emotional disorder caused by emotions of fear and terror. The *Nei Jing (Yellow Emperor's Canon of Internal Medicine)* discusses emotional disorders' impact on the five Zang Organ. It says: The emotion of the Liver is anger; excessive anger will damage the Liver. The emotion of the Kidneys is terror, excessive terror will damage the Kidneys.

Etiology, pathogenesis, and therapy

Horror damages the Kidneys, and Kidney water fails to nourish the Liver resulting in disordered cooperation of the Liver. Additionally, if the Kidney water fails to nourish the Heart it will result in the Heart failing to properly house the Shen leading to PTSD. Generally speaking, PTSD relates to the Heart, Liver and Kidney.

Liver Qi stagnation

Physical and mental stress are common mechanisms leading to Liver Qi stagnation. The Covid-19 pandemic has created massive global stress for people. Healthcare workers, first responders, family members and patients all face unique elements of stress under these conditions. However, what they have in common is that high levels of stress, especially for protracted periods of time will overwhelm the Liver's function of controlling the smooth flow of Qi in the body. When this is disrupted Liver Qi stagnation will occur. Depending on the person's lifestyle and constitution will determine what other organ systems may also be affected.

Manifestations: depression, unrest, grief and sorrow, emotional breakdown, rib-side pain, irregular period, sighing, abdominal bloating, thin tongue coating, wiry pulse on the left and deep and weak on the right.

Treatment strategy: Soothe the Liver Qi and relieve Qi stagnation

Formula: Si Ni San.

For significant Qi stagnation, add Xiang Fu, Chuan Xiong, Qing Pi, Fo Shou. Add Chen Pi, Ban Xia. For burping, acid regurgitation. For Qi stagnation turning to heat with impatience and irritability, Jia Wei Xiao Yao San is used.

Acupuncture points: PC6, Liv3, Sp6, UB17, UB18, St36.

For Qi stagnation turning fire, add GB34, Ki1.

Heart and Spleen deficiency

When Liver Qi stagnation is present, it is common for this stagnant Qi to disable other organ systems' functions. When stagnant Liver Qi disrupts the Spleen and Heart function emotional instability can easily occur. The Spleen makes the blood, the Heart moves the blood and houses the Shen. The Shen relies on Heart blood for anchoring and nourishment. Liver Qi stagnation creates disorder in the Heart/Spleen blood relationship. When Heart blood fails to nourish the Shen, emotional disorders will occur.

Manifestations: terror, insomnia with nightmares that relates to Covid-19, dizziness, fatigue and poor appetite. Pale tongue, deep and weak pulse.

Treatment strategy: supplement the Spleen and Heart, generate blood and calm the mind.

Formula: Gui Pi Tang.

For irritability, add Zhen Zhu Mu, Mu Li. For depression, add He Huan Pi, Ye Jiao Teng. For spontaneous sweating, add Fu Xiao Mai, Duan Mu Li. With Yin and blood deficiency, add Bai He, Mai Men Dong, Wu Wei Zi.

Acupuncture points: UB15, UB20, HT7, Yintang.

For significant fatigue, add ST36, SP6, Du20. For poor sleep, add Anmian, Si Shen Chong.

Heat phlegm disturbing Heart

Stress due to Covid-19 causes Qi stagnation, Qi stagnation turns to heat, the heat burns body fluids and creates phlegm. The heat and phlegm accumulate and disturbs the Heart-mind.

Manifestations: being easily startled or frightened, fear, anxiety, irritability, restlessness, poor sleep, poor appetite, acid regurgitation, red tongue with yellow greasy coating, slippery and rapid pulse.

Treatment strategy: Clear heat and resolve phlegm, relieve restlessness.

Formula: Huang Lian Wen Dan Tang.

For restlessness, add Suan Zao Ren, Yuan Zhi, Long Gu, Mu Li. For Yin deficiency, add Mai Men Dong, Bai He, Zhi Mu.

Acupuncture points: UB15, UB19, PC6, UB23.

For significant fear, add UB45, UB48. For rib-side pain, add SJ6, GB34. For insomnia, add HT7, Anmian. For Yin deficiency, add KI3, UB23.

Heart and Kidney deficiency

Excessive terror will damage the Kidneys. Patients who are suddenly shocked by witnessing or hearing about a death from Covid-19 may experience this shock, the sudden terror injures the Kidneys. Kidney Yin fails to nourish the Heart Yin or Kidney Yang fails to warm the Heart Yang, resulting in both deficiency of Heart and Kidney.

Manifestations: tends to be frightened, palpitations, poor sleep, incontinence of urine or feces after being scared, low back pain and knee pain, low libido. Red tongue with less coating and thin, thready and rapid pulse if it is Kidney Yin deficiency. Pale and swollen tongue with watery coating, deep and weak pulse if it is Yang deficiency.

Treatment Strategy: Supplement Heart and Kidney, sedate the terror.

Formula: Jin Gui Shen Qi Wan for Yang deficiency of the Heart and Kidney. Liu Wei Ji Huang Wan for Yin deficiency of the Heart and Kidney.

For Yang Qi deficiency, add Ren Shen, Long Gu, Mu Li. For deficient heat, add E Jiao, Zhi Mu and Zhen Zhu Mu.

Acupuncture points: UB15, DU4, UB23, Si Shen Chong.

For Yang deficiency, add moxa at UB15 and Du4. For Yang Qi deficiency of the Heart and Kidney Yang, add ST36, Ren12. For Yin deficiency of the Heart and Kidney, add KI3, SP6.

Additional Therapies

Ear acupuncture: Heart, subcortical, Shen Men, forehead, Brain Stem.

Cupping: the UB14, UB15, UB45, UB52.

Exercise: Do Tai Ji, Qi Gong, Yoga.

Spleen and Stomach Injury Post Covid-19

Gastrointestinal sequelae of COVID-19 including loss of appetite, nausea, acid reflux, and diarrhea are common in patients 3 months after discharge from hospital due to COVID-19. Most of the manifestations are related to the Spleen and Stomach in TCM. Persistent gastrointestinal symptoms have important implications for proper management of patients and health-care resources.

Gastrointestinal sequelae were defined as gastrointestinal symptoms that presented after discharge but were not present within the month before onset of COVID-19. There are 44% of patients that reported gastrointestinal symptoms after discharge at the 90 day telephone interview. The most common gastrointestinal sequelae in 117 patients were loss of appetite (24%), nausea (18%), acid reflux (18%), and diarrhea (15%); less common gastrointestinal sequelae included abdominal distension (14%), belching (10%), vomiting (9%), abdominal pain (7%), and bloody stools (2%)[1]. Acupuncture and moxibustion may play a role in the prevention, treatment and rehabilitation of the COVID-19, and relieve the symptoms caused by COVID-19. Acupuncture has been demonstrated to effectively relieve common symptoms in supportive and palliative care, including nausea, insomnia, fatigue as well as vomiting [2][3].

Etiology, pathogenesis and therapy

The manifestations of gastrointestinal sequelae of COVID-19, such as loss of appetite, loss of taste, nausea, acid reflux and diarrhea, are related to the Spleen and Stomach disorders in TCM. The Spleen and Stomach are localized in the middle Jiao and belong to the earth phase. The Spleen belong to Yin earth, it likes dryness and dislikes moisture. The Spleen governs the transporting and transforming of food, which depends on the ascending function of the Spleen. So it is said that the Spleen is in normal condition if it can ascend. The Spleen produces the Qi and blood and ascends the clear Qi and nourishes the whole body. It is the acquired foundation and the source of Qi and blood. The Stomach belongs to Yang earth. It likes moisture and dislikes dryness. The Stomach governs receiving and digestion of food. It is the sea of food which depends on the descending function of the Stomach. So it is said that the Stomach is harmonious when it can descend. If the Spleen and Stomach are injured by COVID-19 virus, or incorrect treatment during COVID-19, the functions of the Spleen and Stomach fail to transform and transport the Qi, there will be disharmony between ascending and descending, resulting in the loss of appetite, loss of taste, nausea, acid reflux and diarrhea and lost taste of mouth.

Damp cold lingering in the Spleen and Stomach

Dampness and cold can linger in the Spleen and Stomach after COVID-19. Additionally patients who were treated using high dose IV therapies, or excessive amounts of cold and bitter herbs may have cold damage to the Spleen and Stomach, which leads to the disorders of Spleen and Stomach functions, manifested with gastrointestinal sequelae of COVID-19.

Manifestations: poor appetite, loss of taste, abdominal bloating, heavy body, fatigue, pale and swollen tongue with thick white and greasy coating, sluggish pulse.

Treatment Strategy: Warm the middle Jiao, dry the dampness and harmonize Spleen and

Stomach.

Formula: Ping Wei San.

For significant cold, add Gao Liang Jiang. For loss of taste, add Huo Xiang, Zi Su Ye. For Spleen deficiency, add Fu Ling, Bai Zhu. For loss of appetite, add Mu Gua, Sha Ren.

Acupuncture points: Ren12, ST25, ST36, PC6.

For a significant cold, add moxa at Ren12, ST25. For loss of taste, add ST4, Ear mouth. For Spleen deficiency, add UB20, UB21. For loss of appetite, add SP4, LI4.

Damp heat lingering the Spleen and Stomach

Damp-heat pathologies can remain in the body during and after COVID-19 infection. Or damp-cold may transform to damp-heat due to long-term stagnation. Incorrect treatment, such as over use of steroids and hot herbal formulas, leads to damp-heat accumulating in the Spleen and Stomach, manifesting with digestive sequelae of COVID-19.

Manifestations: abdominal bloating, acid regurgitation with a foul odor, thirst without desire to drink water, diarrhea, swelling and edema, a red and swollen tongue with a yellow, greasy coating.

Treatment Strategy: clear heat, eliminate dampness, transform the Spleen and Stomach.

Formula: San Ren Tang.

For significant abdominal bloating, add Zhi Shi, Mu Xiang. For significant acid regurgitation, add Zhu Ru, Duan Mu Li. For obvious odor, add Pei Lan, Huo Xiang. For severe diarrhea, add Ge Gen Qin Lian Tang.

Acupuncture points: LI11, SP9, SP4, ST25.

For significant abdominal bloating, add ST36, ST40. For significant acid regurgitation, add Ren12, LIV13. For obvious odor, add ST44, ST4. For severe diarrhea, add SP6, UB25.

Spleen deficiency with dampness accumulation

When Spleen Qi is injured by COVID-19, dampness can linger in the Spleen. The Spleen then fails to transport and transform the foods, resulting in symptoms of COVID-19 sequelae.

Manifestations: diarrhea with indigestion, poor appetite, loss of taste, fatigue, pale, swollen and tender tongue with white, greasy coating, a deep and weak pulse.

Treatment Strategy: supplement Spleen, eliminate dampness and benefit Spleen.

Formula: Shen Ling Bai Zhu San.

For significant indigestion, add Shan Zha, Mu Gua. For obvious poor appetite, add Shan Yao, Ge Gen. For significant fatigue, add Chai Hu and Sheng Ma.

Acupuncture points: UB20, UB21, UB25, Ren12.

For significant indigestion, add Inner Nei Ting, Ren9. For obvious poor appetite, add ST36, SP4. For significant fatigue, add DU20 and ST36.

Spleen Yang deficiency

Patients with pre-existing Spleen deficiency before COVID-19 infection, will suffer further Spleen damage and especially Spleen Yang. In addition, patients who have used excessive amounts of cold, bitter and purgative herbs will likely damage Spleen Yang manifesting the symptoms of COVID-19 sequelae.

Manifestations: Dull abdominal pain, watery diarrhea, poor appetite, vomiting, fatigue, cold extremities with edema, a pale and swollen tongue with watery coating, and a deep and weak pulse.

Treatment Strategy: Warm the Spleen and supplement Qi, stop pain and diarrhea.

Formula: Xiao Jian Zhong Tang or Li Zhong Wan.

For dull abdominal pain due to Spleen Qi and blood deficiency, choose Xiao Jian Zhong Tang. For chronic diarrhea due to Spleen Yang deficiency and cold, choose Li Zhong Wan. For edema and cold extremities add Fu Zi, Rou Gui.

Acupuncture points: REN 12, REN8, ST36, SP6.

For warming Yang, add moxa at Ren8 and Ren12. For abdominal pain, add ST25 with moxa. For vomiting, add PC6, SP4.

Reference:

1. Jingrong Weng, Yichen Li, Jie Li, et al. Gastrointestinal sequelae 90 days after discharge for COVID-19. *Lancet Gastroenterol Hepatol.* 2021 May;6(5):344-346. doi: 10.1016/S2468-1253(21)00076-5. Epub 2021 Mar 10.
2. Vn Trott P, Oei SL, Ramsenthaler C. Acupuncture for breathlessness in advanced diseases: a systematic review and meta-analysis. *J Pain Symptom Manage* 2020;59:327.e3–38.e3.
3. Amorim D, Amado J, Brito I, et al. Acupuncture and electroacupuncture for anxiety disorders: a systematic review of the clinical research. *Complement Ther Clin Pract* 2018;31:31–7.

Heart Function Injury Post Covid-19

Clinical studies suggest that COVID-19 is associated with a high incidence of cardiac arrhythmias. Severe acute respiratory syndrome coronavirus infection may cause injury to cardiac myocytes and increase arrhythmia risk. There are well-documented cardiac complications of COVID-19 in patients with and without prior cardiovascular disease. There is growing evidence showing that arrhythmias are also one of the major complications.

In TCM, arrhythmia is discussed in palpitation (Xin Ji 心悸) and panic attack (Jing Kong, 惊恐), it refers to the unduly rapid Heartbeat which is felt by the patient and accompanied by nervousness, feelings of fear, restlessness, insomnia, forgetfulness and dizziness.

Dr Xue Shengbai in his book, *the Damp warm febrile disease* (27th section) says "The damp warm disease is treated following other therapies. If after all of the other symptoms have disappeared, the patient still has palpitations and nightmares, this is due to lingering evils still inside and results in Gallbladder stagnation". Dr. Wu Tang in his book, *Systemic Differentiation of Warm Pathogen Disease* (14th section) says "When there is warm febrile disease in the lower Jiao, the heat is deep and severe, which causes the patient to suffer from thin, rapid and irregular pulse, severe palpitation in the chest, and even chest pain. The formula is San Jia Fu Mai Tang (Three Shells for Recovering pulse decoction)". In the 11th section of his book he also says "when there are warm febrile diseases in the Shaoyin, the true Yin tends to be exhausted, the deficient fire burns the Heart, resulting in anxiety and insomnia. Huang Lian E Jiao Tang is good for it".

Etiology, pathogenesis and therapy

Covid-19 depletes Qi, blood, Yin and Yang of the Heart, which is the root cause of palpitations in post Covid-19 patients, and leads to the accumulation of phlegm and body fluids, Qi stagnation, blood stasis, and heat and fire lingering in the Heart; these are the branch symptoms of post Covid-19 palpitations.

Qi and Blood deficiency of the Heart

There are several mechanisms leading to Heart Qi and blood deficiency. These include the pathogens of Covid-19 lingering inside and overtreatment of Covid-19. All of these damage Qi and blood to the Spleen and Heart.

Manifestations: palpitation, shortness of breath, easy to be frightened, poor sleep and memory, restlessness, sweating at palms, pale tongue with white and thin coating, deep, weak, knotted and intermittent pulse.

Treatment Strategy: reinforce Qi and blood of Spleen and Heart, calm the mind.

Formula: Gui Pi Tang

For significant palpitations and an irregular pulse add Zhi Gan Cao Tang. If there are feelings of fear add Long Gu and Mu Li.

Acupuncture points: PC6, UB15, UB17, St36, UB20.

Heart Yang deficiency

The lingering dampness due to Covid-19 and overuse of medicine or other therapies to treat Covid-19 consumes the Heart Yang and fails to warm the Heart.

Manifestations: palpitations that are worse with activity, chest fullness, cold extremities, edema of the lower legs, pale face. The tongue body is white with a wet coating, the pulse is deep and weak.

Treatment Strategy: Warm and tonify the Heart Yang, calm the Heart spirit.

Formula: Gui Zhi Jia Long Gu Mu Li Tang

For significant Heart Yang deficiency, add Ren Shen and Fu Zi. If accompanied by Yin

deficiency, add Mai Men Dong, Bai He and Wu Wei Zi. For significant fullness of the chest, edema

of the legs use Ling Gui Zhu Gan Tang.

Acupuncture points: Ht 7, PC6, UB15(moxa), Ren17(moxa). For Qi deficiency, add St36,

Ren12.

Heart fire due to Yin depletion

High fever, or excessive sweating injures the Heart and Yin resulting in Heart fire. The deficient fire disturbs the Heart spirit.

Manifestations: palpitations and anxiousness, nervousness and anxiety, poor sleep, nightmares, hot sensation of the five palms, dizziness, red face, soreness of low back, red tongue with less coating, thin and rapid pulse.

Treatment strategy: Supplement Yin and clear heat, nourish Heart and calm spirit.

Formula: Huang Lian E Jiao Tang

For nervousness and anxiety, add Suan Zao Ren and Mu Li. For soreness of the low back and hot flashes, add Huang Bai and Zhi Mu. For mild heat use Tian Wang Bu Xin Dan.

Acupuncture points: Ht7, PC6, Ki6, UB23. For anxiety, add Yintang, Si Shen Chong, and Ear Shen Men. For soreness of low back and hot flash, add Sp6, Ear Jian.

Heat phlegm disturbing Heart

The lingering heat after Covid-19 burns the fluids of the Lung, transforming into hot phlegm, which disturbs the Heart.

Manifestations: frequent palpitations, easy to be scared, chest fullness, anxiety, insomnia, nightmares, thirst, constipation, red tongue with yellow greasy coating, slippery and wiry pulse.

Treatment strategy: Clear heat and resolve phlegm, tranquilize the Heart mind.

Formula: Huang Lian Wen Dan Tang

Add Zhi Zi, Gua Lou, Suan Zao Ren to clear heat and resolve phlegm. For significant anxiety, add Shi Jue Ming and Zhen Zhu Mu. When heat and fire injure Yin, add Mai Men Dong and Yu Zhu.

Acupuncture points: Ht4, PC4, Lu5, Lu10.

Blood stasis blocking Heart

Heart Qi and blood deficiency post Covid 19 weaken Qi and it fails to move the blood. Heat phlegm blocks the Heart vessels. All of these result in blood stasis blocking the Heart vessels.

Manifestations: palpitations and anxiety, chest distress and stabbing pain, purple tongue and choppy or knotted pulse.

Treatment strategy: Regulate Qi and remove blood stasis, open meridian.

Formula: Xue Fu Zhu Yu Tang.

For blood stasis due to Yang deficiency and cold, add Gui Zhi and Fu Zi. For significant Qi stagnation, add Tan Xiang and Qing Pi. For damp-phlegm with fullness of the chest, add Gua Lou, Xie Bai and Ban Xia.

Acupuncture points: PC3, Ht3, Sp10, Ren6.

Additional therapies

Ear points: Ht, sympathetic, subcortical, Small Intestine.

Cupping: Ren 17, Ren14, UB14, UB15.

Liver Function Injury Post Covid-19

Unusual Liver enzyme levels are a common finding in COVID-19 patients. Usually, it is seen in the form of altered aminotransferases picked up during routine blood tests. The cause of the Liver injury is not clearly established, but most likely, it seems multifactorial, with a cytokine storm and immune dysregulation possibly playing a role so it could be hypoxia, hypotension, multiple drugs, direct viral effect, and ICU-related infections. There data indicate that 2–11% of patients with COVID-19 showed Liver comorbidities and 14–53% cases reported abnormal levels of alanine aminotransferase and aspartate aminotransferase (AST) during disease progression. Patients with severe COVID-19 infection seem to have higher rates of Liver dysfunction. [1]

Furthermore, another study showed Liver injury is more prevalent in severe cases than in mild cases of COVID-19. AST abnormal 22·2%, ALT abnormal 21·3% [2].

The Liver injury may manifest as jaundice, rib-side pain, fatigue, low grade fever. However, abnormally elevated transferases are one of the most common issues. TCM therapies have been used to help treat Liver disorders effectively. Based on the presentation, the post Covid-19 Liver damage pattern can be referred to Jaundice and rib-side pain in TCM. The *Shang Han Lun says,* "Exterior cold exists simultaneously with interior heat which surely leads to jaundice". The *Golden Chamber on Jaundice says,* "Jaundice is due to dampness". Dr Ye Gui in his book, *Case Records as a Guide to Clinical Practice on Jaundice* says, "treat the Stomach for Yang jaundice, treat the Spleen for Yin jaundice". Since then, many effective TCM formulas and acupuncture therapies have been used for improving Liver enzymes.

Etiology, Pathogenesis and Therapy

The turbid dampness component of Covid-19 lingers inside long term and turns to heat. Dampness and heat mix and invade the Liver and Gallbladder resulting in disharmony of Liver and Gallbladder. The bile is forced out abnormally and the Liver function is injured by the damp-heat, manifesting as raised Liver transaminases and Yang Jaundice. Moreover, the dampness of Covid-19 may turn to cold. Damp- cold accumulates in the Spleen, blocking Liver Qi and resulting in elevated Liver enzymes. The bile is blocked, and the bile moves abnormally resulting in jaundice.

Damp heat in the Liver and Gallbladder

Damp heat aspects of Covid-19 not only invade the Lung, but also affect the Liver and Gallbladder.

Manifestations: Liver AST and ALT increase rapidly, yellow sclera, rib-side fullness and pain, low grade fever, poor appetite, red tongue with yellow greasy coating, wiry pulse.

Treatment strategy: soothe the Liver and clear heat, resolve dampness, and decrease transaminases.

Formula: Yin Chen Hao Tang.

If there is severe dampness and heat add Long Dan Xie Gan Tang. For significant

abnormal Liver transaminases, add Wu Wei Zi, Gan Huang Cao, Chui Peng Cao. For dampness, add

Fu Ling and Zhu Ling. For nausea, vomiting, add Zhu Ru and Chen Pi. For high heat and a thick, yellow greasy tongue coating, add Huang Bai, Huang Qin.

Acupuncture points: GB34, LV13, SP9, UB19, REN12.

For nausea, vomiting, add PC6, UB20. For heat, add LI11 and ST44.

Liver Qi stagnation

Resentment, frustration, and the stress with Covid-19 can cause stagnation of Liver Qi, which disrupts the soothing function of the Liver and leads to elevated Liver transaminases. Over time, the stagnation of Liver qi may give rise to Liver stasis and/or Liver heat.

Manifestations: mental depression, bile secretion disorders, poor digestion, menstrual irregularities

Treatment strategy: Regulate Liver Qi, harmonize the Liver function.

Formula: Xiao Yao San

For Qi stagnation turning to heat, add Mu Dan Pi, Zhi Zi. For Qi stagnation with blood stasis, add Dan Shen, Yu Jin.

Acupuncture points: LV3, LI4, Ren6, SP6.

For heat, add DU14, LI11. For blood stasis, add SP10, UB17.

Spleen deficiency and damp accumulation

The consumption of Spleen Yang post Covid-19 or the exterior damp-cold of Covid-19 can linger inside. This leads to the formation of damp-cold in the Spleen and damage of the Liver and Gallbladder functions, which blocks bile resulting in jaundice.

Manifestations: chronic abnormal Liver transaminases, dull jaundice and rib-side pain, fatigue, poor appetite, loose stool, loss of taste, pale tongue with white and greasy coating, sluggish pulse.

Treatment strategy: Strengthen the Spleen and Stomach, warm interior, resolve dampness, decrease transaminases.

Formula: Yin Chen Zhu Fu Tang.

For elevated transaminases, may add Shan Zha, Mu Gua, Wu Wei Zi, Gan Huang Cao. For fullness of

abdomen, add Hou Po, Cang Zhu. For loss of taste add Huo Xiang and Zi Su Ye.

Acupuncture points: ST36, SP6, Ren4(Moxa), LV13.

For fullness of the abdomen, add ST25, Ren12. For tasteless, add SP4, Ear tongue.

Liver Blood Stasis

The Liver Qi stagnation, damp-heat or cold of long term Covid-19 may give rise to blood stasis resulting in injured Liver function.

Manifestations: abnormal Liver transaminases that are difficult to be helped, stabbing and fixed hypochondrial pain, feeling of a mass of palpation, purple tongue with choppy or wiry.

Treatment strategy: Soothe the Liver, move Qi and blood, improve the Liver transaminases.

Formula: Chai Hu Su Gan San.

For significant blood stasis, add Dan Shen, Jiang Huang. For significantly elevated Liver transaminases, add Hu Zhang, Gan Huang Cao. For rib-side pain, add Yu Jin, Tao Ren.

Acupuncture points: LV3, LV5, SP21, UB17.

For blood stasis, add SP10, LV King. For hypochondrial pain, add LV13.

Additional Therapies

Ear points: Gallbladder, Liver, Spleen, Stomach.

Patent herbs:

Gan Su Jiao Nang (Recovering Liver Capsules): it is used for abnormal Liver transaminases due to damp- heat in Liver and Gallbladder. 2 capsules per time, 3 times per day.

Fu Fang Yi Gan Pian (Complex Strengthen Liver Pills): it is used for abnormal Liver transaminases. 4 pills per time, 3 times per day.

Chui Pen Cao Granules (Herba Sedi Powder): it is used for abnormal Liver transaminases. 10g per time, 3 times per day.

Reference:

1. Chao Zhang, Lei Shi, Fu-Sheng Wang. Ler Injury in Covid-19: Management and Challenges The Lancet Gastroenterology & Hepatology. March 04, 2020.

Guan W-J, Ni Z-Y, Hu Yet al.Clinical characteristics of 2019 novel coronavirus infection in China.*N Engl J Med.* 2020.

Lung Function Injury Post Covid-19

Many patients after having Covid-19 have shortness of breath, dry and hacking cough, aching joints and muscles. These symptoms are related to post-inflammatory pulmonary fibrosis (PPF). Most COVID-19 patients were having PPF on the follow-up CT scan when discharged and complaining about exertional dyspnea of different levels. Medical studies have shown that 70% of patients who were infected with common Covid-19 develop PPF and in patients who suffered severe infections, PPF was present 100% of the time. Traditional Chinese medicine and rehabilitation may also help the Lung function injury post Covid-19.

In TCM, the PPF might be referred to Lung Atrophy (肺痿Fei Wei) and/ or Lung Distention (肺胀Fei Zhang). The *Golden Chamber* says: Heat in the upper Jiao manifests as cough resulting in Lung atrophy.

Etiology, pathogenesis, and therapy

Chronic cough, dampness and heat which are common mechanisms of Covid-19 injures and burns the Lung Yin. The Lungs fail to be nourished and over time can develop into Lung atrophy. Chronic cough can lead to Qi deficiency which weakens the physical constitution and consumes the Qi and Yang of Lung, Spleen and Kidney. Yang Qi deficiency results in the failure to metabolize fluids, therefore the Lungs are not nourished leading to Lung atrophy.

Turbid phlegm accumulates in the Lung, this phlegm can linger on long term and result in deficiency of Spleen and Kidney. Disorders of the Lungs, Spleen and Kidney ultimately injure the hHart and Liver function. Qi deficiency and phlegm block the Lung's function of depurative downbearing leading to blood stasis, as well as phlegm and blood stasis obstructing Lung Qi. Qi and Yin deficiency are at the root of Covid-19, damp phlegm and blood stasis are branches of Covid-19 infection.

Yin deficiency and phlegm sticky in the Lung

Damp-heat lingers in the Lungs after Covid-19 infection injuring the Lung Yin from chronic cough. This can also occur due to improper treatment or extended use of acrid and hot herbs. Ultimately the Lungs fail in their descending function because of damaged Lung Yin. This manifests as severe cough, wheezing, and dry throat. The interior heat burns the Lung fluid creating phlegm and presenting as cough with sticky and frothy sputum.

Manifestations: cough and wheezing with sticky and frothy sputum, blood in the phlegm, thirst, dry mouth, fever that is worse in the afternoon, thin body and dry skin. Red and dry tongue, weak and rapid pulse.

Treatment Strategy: Clear heat and nourish the Lung Yin.

Formula: Mai Men Dong Tang.

For Lung Yin deficiency with significant dry heat, use Qing Zhao Jiu Fei Tang. For significantly injured Yin, add Sha Shen, Yu Zhu. For copious sticky and yellow phlegm due to phlegm heat, add Chuan Bei Mu, Tian Hua Fen. For hot flashes due to Yin deficiency, add Yin Chai Hu and Di Gu Pi. For Qi and Yin deficiency of the Lungs, add Sheng Mai San.

Acupuncture points: UB13, UB23, Lu7, Lu10, Ki3. For significant Yin deficiency, add UB23, Ki6.

Lung Qi deficiency with phlegm accumulating in the Lung

The Spleen is the original organ that produces phlegm, and the Lung stores the phlegm. When cold phlegm is stored in the Lungs, it manifests as cough with copious watery and frothy sputum, a lower voice and shortness of breath.

Manifestations: cough with copious watery and frothy sputum, lower voice and shortness of breath, dizziness and fatigue, cold extremities, poor appetite, profuse urine, pale tongue, deep and weak pulse.

Treatment Strategy: Generate the Qi and warm the Lungs

Formula: Gan Cao Gan Jiang Tang.

For significant Spleen Qi deficiency, add Fu Ling and Bai Zhu. For shortness of breath, and weak voice, add Huang Qi and Wu Wei Zi. For significant phlegm, add Jin Shui Liu Jun Jian, it uses Dang Gui, Shu Di Huang, Chen Pi, Ban Xia, Fu Ling and Zhi Gan Cao for both deficiency of Lung and Kidney.

Acupuncture points: Lu1, UB13, Du4(moxa), Ren6(moxa), Ki6. For significant phlegm accumulating in the Lungs, add St40, Ren22.

Heat and toxin obstructing in the Lung

Heat and toxins of a Covid-19 infection linger in the Lungs, scorching fluids leading to dampness and phlegm accumulation which, in turn, injures the Lungs' vessels, manifesting as cough with a foul odor and bleeding.

Manifestations: cough with yellow sputum, fever, chest pain, shortness of breath, thirst, red tongue with yellow greasy coating and slippery rapid pulse.

Treatment Strategy: clear heat from Lung, transform phlegm, drive out blood stasis.

Formula: Wei Jing Tang.

For significant heat toxins in the Lungs with yellow or green sputum, add Jie Jeng, Yu Xing Cao, Pu Gong Ying to clear toxins and discharge pus. With high fever and anxiety, add Huang Qin, Huang Lian, Zhi Zi, Jin Yin Hua.

Acupuncture point: St44, Lu7, Ren17, L11, PC6.

Phlegm and blood stasis blocking Lung

Dampness formed from a Covid-19 infection can remain in the Lungs and lead to Lung Yin deficiency, and Qi deficiency of Lungs and Spleen. This can lead to blood becoming sluggish blocking the Lungs, leading to more phlegm and blood stasis. This manifests as a cough with purple blood in the sputum.

Manifestations: cough and wheezing with purple blood in the sputum, shortness of breath, chest pain, palpitation, purple extremities, lips and tongue, watery coating, deep and choppy pulse.

Treatment Strategy: Supplement Qi and invigorate blood, resolve phlegm and open Lung Qi.

Formula: Bu Yang Huan Wu Tang and Bu Fei Tang.

Bu Yang Huang Wu Tang is used for blood stasis due to Qi deficiency. Huang Qi, Ren Shen and Wu Wei Zi strongly supplement the Lungs, Spleen and Heart Qi. Dang Gui, Chuan Xiong, Chi Shao, Di Long, Tao Ren and Hong Hua invigorate blood and expel the vessels blocking Lung and Heart Qi. Shu Di Huang, Wu Wei Zi also strengthen the Kidney essence and assist the Lung Qi's downbearing function. Zi Wan, Sang Bai Pi and Tao Ren resolve the phlegm to stop coughing. For significant phlegm in the Lung, add Ban Xia, Zhe Bei Mu, Xing Ren.

Acupuncture points: Lu1, UB17, PC6, Ki6, St36, Ren17. For significant phlegm, add St40, Ren22

Additional Therapies

Cupping: Cup UB13, UB14, UB15, UB17.

Guasha: Push Guasha along the Du and UB channel from UB12 to UB17.

Xue Wei Tie Fu (herbal patch to place on acupuncture points): Ingredients: Ren Shen, Wu Wei Zi, Bai Jie Zi and Tao Ren is 10g. Grind each into powder and use 0.5g of each, put on each point at UB14, UB17. It is used for PPF due to Qi deficiency with blood stasis blocking in the Lung vessels.

Renal Injury Post Covid -19

A new comprehensive report shows that up to 30% of patients hospitalized with COVID-19 in China and New York developed moderate or severe Kidney injury. Reports from doctors in New York are saying the percentage could be higher (https://www.hopkinsmedicine.org/health/conditions-and-diseases/coronavirus/coronavirus-Kidney-damage-caused-by-covid19). The Kidney damage is, in some cases, severe enough to require dialysis. Some hospitals experiencing surges of patients who are very ill with COVID-19 have reported they are running short on the machines and sterile fluids needed to perform these Kidney procedures.

Signs of Kidney problems in patients with COVID-19 include high levels of protein in the urine and abnormal blood work. According to the manifestations of the renal injury post Covid-19, it can be referred to Shui Zhong (Edema), Xue Niao (Bleeding urine), Niao Zhuo (Cloudy urine) or Long Bi (Oliguria and anuria) in TCM. The *Huang Di Nei Jing · Chapter 61 Shui Re Xue Lun says*: The Kidney is like the sluice gate of the Stomach, when the sluice gate does not work, the fluid will be accumulated and the evils will run wild, when the fluid overflows about the skin, peritoneal fluid will occur. As the spreading of the Kidney Qi and the Lung Qi are correlated with each other, the retention of fluid will cause both viscera to suffer disease. The root of edema is in the Kidney and its symptoms are manifested in the Lungs. The book also points out the therapeutic principle for edema is to perspire and promote urination. The *Golden Chamber* on Edema mentions there are four edemas; they are Wind edema, Skin edema, Zheng Edema and Shi Edema. The therapeutic principle of edema is to promote urine for all edema below the waist and promote sweating with edema above the waist. Zhu Bing Yuan Hou Lun (General Treatise on the Causes and Symptoms of Diseases) says: Edema are due to deficiency of the Spleen and Kidney.

Etiology, pathogenesis, and therapy

The Lungs, Spleen and Kidney play key roles in Kidney injury post covid-19. When covid-19 invades the Lungs, the opening and closing of the pores is disrupted and this leads to a failure of regulating the water ways. Therefore, the water accumulates under the skin, resulting in edema. If the toxic heat of covid-19 directly attacks the Kidneys and burns the Kidney vessels it will result in abnormal levels of protein in the urine and blood in the hematuria. Improper treatment or long-term Covid infection damages the Spleen and Kidney. The weak Spleen fails to lift the essence, the weak Kidney fails to store essence and the essence leaks out.

Virus in the Lung, wind water under skin

Covid-19 invades the body from the exterior, stagnating the exterior, the Lungs fail to open and close the pores which regulate the water ways. The water accumulates under the skin, manifesting as edema. If the Lung Qi is inhibited by the virus, clear Qi from the Spleen fails to ascend to the Lungs and moves downward abnormally, resulting in proteinuria.

Manifestations: puffy and edema that is worse at upper body, urinal protein or urinal bleeding, oliguria, chills, fever, aching body, no sweating, cough or shortness of breath, white coating, floating tight pulse.

Treatment Strategy: expel wind and relieve exterior, disperse the Lungs, and promote urination.

Formula: Ma Huang Lian Qiao Chi Xiao Dou Tang, Wu Wei Xiao Du Yin.

In this formula, Fu Ping is used to replace Ma Huang. For significant edema, increase the dose of Fu Ping from 9g to 15g. For protein in urine, add Yu Xing Cao, Lu Gen. For hematuria, add Bai Mao Gen, Xiao Ji. For significant edema, add Zhu Ling, Ze Xie. For sore throat, add Niu Bang Zi, Ban Lan Gen. For cough and shortness of breath, add Xing Ren, Sang Bai Pi.

Acupuncture points: LU5, SJ5, UB22, UB13.

For proteinuria, add REN3. For hematuria, add UB17. For sore throat, add LU10.

Heat toxin damaging Lung and Kidney

The heat toxin of Covid-19 attacks the Lungs and Kidneys directly. The overuse of medicine, herbs and other therapies may also injure the Kidney function.

Manifestations: Acute poor Kidney function, urinal protein and bleeding, sores or purpura around all body, less urine and edema, red tongue with yellow greasy coating, deep rapid pulse.

Treatment Strategy: clear heat and eliminate dampness, reduce protein and stop bleeding.

Formula: Si Miao San, Xiao Jie Yin Zi, Hua Ban Tang.

For reddish sores with pus, add Huang Lian Jie Du Tang. For hematuria, use Xiao Jie Yin Zi. For significant purpura, use Hua Ban Tang. For acute renal failure, add Da Huang, Dan Shen.

Acupuncture points: REN9, DU14, UB40, SP10.

For reddish sores or purpura, bleeding UB40, add ST44. With decreased urine, add UB39, UB23.

Dampness accumulating in the Spleen

Patients with Covid-19 are given IV fluid. Due to the IV fluid infusion's cold thermal properties overtaking of cold herbs, the virus damaging the Spleen directly all leads to damp accumulation in the Spleen. Therefore, the Spleen fails to transport and transform food and fluids, resulting in water retention under the skin as edema.

Manifestations: puffy extremities, proteinuria, heavy body, nausea, poor appetite, loose stool, pale and swollen tongue with white greasy coating, deep sluggish pulse.

Treatment Strategy: Strengthen the Spleen and eliminate dampness, promote urination and reduce edema.

Formula: Wei Ling Tang

For Spleen Qi deficiency, add Dang Shen and Huang Qi. For less urine, add Che Qian Zi, Sang Bai Pi. For proteinuria add Huang Qi, Yi Yi Ren.

Acupuncture points: UB21, SP9, ST36, SP6.

For Spleen and Stomach deficiency, add REN12, UB21. For less urine, add UB39, UB28. For proteinuria, add REN4, DU20.

The Yang deficiency of both Spleen and Kidney

The Spleen is the root of postnatal Qi and the source of Qi and blood production. Covid-19 directly invades the Spleen and Kidney, or the Spleen and Kidney Yang are injured by improper treatment of Covid-19. When the Kidney function is severely injured, it results in water retention and edema due to both Spleen and Kidney deficiency. Both organs fail to store essence, resulting in proteinuria.

Manifestations: severe renal function injured, pitting edema in all body, puffy eyes' lips, ascites, pleural effusion, pale complexion, fatigue, cold extremities, poor appetite, cough and shortness of breath and difficulty lying down, pale and swollen tongue with slippery and white coating, deep and weak pulse.

Treatment Strategy: warm the Yang and promote urination.

Formula: Zhen Wu Tang.

For Spleen or Heart Qi deficiency and proteinuria, add Ren Shen and Huang Qi. For dampness, add Wu Ling San. For Kidney Yang deficiency, add Rou Gui and Ba Ji Tian.

Acupuncture points: UB20, DU4, SP9, REN4.

For Yang deficiency, add moxa at above points. For Spleen deficiency, add ST36, Ren12.

Qi stagnation and blood stasis

During Covid-19 infection Yin is damaged and increases viscosity of the blood and slows down blood circulation leading to blood stasis. Finally, the blood stasis may turn into water retention and the water retention also hampers circulation.

Manifestations: dull or dark complexion, stubborn urinal protein, stubborn edema or not severe edema, sore lower back, continues bleeding in urine, purple tongue, choppy pulse.

Treatment Strategy: invigorate blood, improve Kidney function.

Formula: Tao Hong Si Wu Tang.

For severe blood stasis, add Qian Cao, San Leng, even Shui Zhi, Di Long. For hematuria, add Pu Huang, Bai Ji. For Qi deficiency, add Dang Shen, Huang Qi.

Acupuncture points: UB17, UB28, SP6, Du4.

For blood stasis, bleed UB17 and SP10. For Yin deficiency, add UB23, KI3.

Additional therapies

Ear points: Ear KI, SP, Ear SHEN MEN.

Patent herbs: Wu Ling San: 6 grams per time, three times per day. It is used for edema due to dampness accumulating in the Spleen.

Liu Wei Di Huang Wan: 6 grams per time, three times per day. It is used for weakness of renal function due to Liver and Kidney deficiency.

Chapter Five

Review of Research on TCM treatment for COVID-19

Coronavirus (COVID-19) is caused by a new coronavirus first identified in Wuhan, China, in December of 2019. Because it is a new virus, scientists are learning more each day. Although most people who have COVID-19 have mild symptoms, COVID-19 can also cause severe illness and even death. Some groups, including older adults and people who have certain underlying medical conditions are at increased risk of severe illness. On February 11, 2020, the World Health Organization announced an official name for the disease that is causing the 2019 novel coronavirus outbreak. The new name of this disease is coronavirus disease 2019, abbreviated as COVID-19. In COVID-19, 'CO' stands for 'corona,' 'VI' for 'virus,' and 'D' for disease. Formerly, this disease was referred to as "2019 novel coronavirus" or "2019-nCoV." (https://www.cdc.gov/coronavirus). COVID-19 is caused by SARS-COV2 and represents the causative agent of a potentially fatal disease that is of great global public health concern.

The initial symptoms of COVID-19 mainly include fever, cough, myalgia, fatigue, or dyspnea. In the later stages of the disease, dyspnea may occur and gradually develop into acute respiratory distress syndrome (ARDS) or multiple organ failure. It has been reported that a cytokine storm is associated with the deterioration of many infectious diseases, including SARS (severe acute respiratory syndrome) and Middle East respiratory syndrome (MERS). The cytokine storm caused by COVID-19 has been suggested to be associated with COVID-19 severity. However, there is currently a limited understanding of the cytokine storm in severe

COVID-19. Therefore, here, we have discussed the current findings and treatment strategies for the cytokine storm in severe COVID-19.

The modern therapies include:

Chloroquine: Delivered in vitro for antiviral effects and anti-inflammatory properties, chloroquine (CQ) and its analog hydroxychloroquine (HCQ) are potential therapies for COVID-19. However, a meta-analysis of clinical trials indicated no clinical benefits of HCQ treatment in patients with COVID-19. In fact, HCQ might actually do more harm than good given its side effects, which include retinopathy, cardiomyopathy, neuromyopathy, and myopathy [1], but some clinical trials have suggested that taking high doses of HCQ or CQ may also cause arrhythmia [2].

Corticosteroids: Given the urgent clinical demand, some experts have recommended the rational use of corticosteroids with severe COVID-19. Although evidence indicates a potential role for the use of corticosteroids in patients with severe COVID-19, caution should be exercised given the possibilities of viral rebound and adverse events [3].

Tocilizumab: Tocilizumab (TCZ), an IL-6 receptor (IL-6R) antagonist, can inhibit cytokine storms by blocking the IL-6 signal transduction pathway. A retrospective case-control study of COVID-19 patients with ARDS revealed that TCZ might improve survival outcomes [4].

Mesenchymal stem cells (MSCs): MSC therapy was found to significantly reduce the mortality of patients with H7N9-induced ARDS. Clinical study of mesenchymal stem cells treating acute respiratory distress syndrome induced by epidemic Influenza A (H7N9) infection, a hint for COVID-19 treatment [5]. Although the side effects of MSC treatment are rarely reported, the safety and effectiveness of this treatment require further investigation.

Most of the above therapies can improve the symptoms of COVID-19, but they also offer multiple side effects with varying severity. Treatment of COVID-19 still needs more research to further verify outcomes. Therefore, it is necessary to find other effective therapies for COVID-19.

Covid-19 and TCM

With COVID-19 spreading rapidly around the globe, traditional medicine also has been widely used for preventing and treating it. After the pandemic happened in Wuhan, China, The COVID-19 patients were treated using Western and traditional Chinese medicine in most hospitals. Most of their academic papers reported significant improvement in approximately 90% of cases. [6]

Traditional Chinese Medicine Therapies include:

Patent Herbs:

Jinhua Qinggan Granule: It was developed during the 2009 H1N1 influenza pandemic. It consists of 12 herbal components including Jin Yin Hua, Shi Gao, Zhi Ma Huang, Xing Ren, Huang Qin, Lian Qiao, Zhe Bei Mu, Zhi Mu, Niu Bang Zi, Qing Hao, Bo He and Gan Cao. It can clear Lung heat and detoxify the Lungs.

It has a curative effect in treating mild and moderate patients and can also improve the recovery rate of lymphocytes and white blood cells as well as reduce the rate of patients turning more severe. A paper reported that among the 80 cases treated with Jin Hua Qing Gan Granule, the average duration of viral nucleic acid detection was (7 ± 4) d in the Jinhua Qinggan administration group and (10 ± 4) d for the control group ($P = 0.010$), following which, nucleic acid tests were negative. Of the two groups, 56.82% in the Jinhua Qinggan treatment group and 27.78% in the control group demonstrated negative nucleic acid tests within 7 days or less. The 7-day viral clearance rate was significantly higher in the Jinhua Qinggan group compared with the control group ($P = 0.009$). Furthermore, the pneumonia recovery time indicated by chest CT was (8 ± 4) d in the Jinhua Qinggan group, which was significantly shorter than the control group, at (10 ± 5) d ($P = 0.021$). No adverse reactions were found in the treatment group after taking this medicine. The author believes that patients with COVID-19, Jinhua Qinggan granules can effectively shorten the duration of nucleic acid detection and promote the absorption of pneumonia inflammatory exudates without obvious adverse reactions [7].

Xuebijing Injection: This injection has Hong Hua, Chi Shao, Chuan Xiong, Dan Shen and Dang Gui. It was developed and marketed during the severe acute respiratory syndrome (SARS) epidemic in 2003. It consists of five herbal extracts and its main function is to detoxify and remove blood stasis. It is usually used to treat sepsis. It is effective in suppressing systemic inflammatory response syndrome induced by infection in the treatment of severe and critically ill patients as well as repairing impaired organ function.

Initial clinical studies have shown that the injection, combined with Western medicine, can increase the rate of hospital discharge and reduce the rate of deterioration. Basic research has also found that it has a certain antiviral effect in vitro that can significantly inhibit inflammatory factors induced by novel coronavirus infection.

The novel coronavirus also tends to cause excessive clotting in the body that leads to organ embolism and damage to tissues, and Xuebijing can help prevent excessive coagulation and the formation of thrombus.

A paper reported 60 cases, the results showed that (1) After treatment, the white blood cell count (WBC) and lymphocyte count (LYM) of three groups increased, meanwhile CRP and ESR decreased. Compared with routine treatment group, the WBC count of Xuebijing 100 mL group after treatment significantly increased ($\times 10^9$/L: 7.12±0.55 vs. 5.67±0.51, $P < 0.05$), and the levels of CRP and ESR in Xuebijing 50 mL and 100 mL groups significantly decreased. Compared with the Xuebijing 50 mL group, the increase of WBC, and the decrease of CRP and ESR were more significant in the Xuebijing 100 mL group. (2) After treatment, the APACHE II score of three groups decreased. In the Xuebijing 100 mL group, the APACHE II score after treatment was significantly lower than those in routine treatment and Xuebijing 50 mL groups ($P < 0.05$). After treatment, the 2019-nCoV nucleic acid test in three groups partly turned negative, with 9 cases in routine treatment group, 8 cases in Xuebijing 50 mL group and 9 cases in Xuebijing 100 mL group, without significant difference ($P > 0.05$). The conditions of patients in the three groups were improved after treatment, among them, 8 cases in the routine treatment group were transformed into common type, 1 case into critical type; 9

cases and 12 cases of Xuebijing 50 mL group and 100 mL group were transformed into common type respectively. Xuebijing 100 mL group was improved more obviously than Xuebijing 50 mL group and routine treatment group (both P < 0.05).

This research showed that Xuebijing injection can effectively improve the inflammatory markers and prognosis of severe COVID-19 patients [8].

Huo Xiang Zheng Qi San: This is a classical formula. It can combine with angiotensin converting enzyme II (ACE2) binding to PTGS2, HSP90AB1, AR, CAMSAP2 and other targets to regulate multiple signaling pathways, thus exerting a preventive or therapeutic effect on COVID-19 [9].

Single Herbs:

Yu Xing Cao: It could stimulate the proliferation of mouse splenic lymphocytes significantly and dose-dependently. By flow cytometry, it was revealed that HC increased the proportion of CD4(+) and CD8(+) T cells. Moreover, it caused a significant increase in the secretion of IL-2 and IL-10 by mouse splenic lymphocytes. In the antiviral aspect, HC exhibited significant inhibitory effects on SARS-CoV 3C-like protease (3CL (pro)) and RNA-dependent RNA polymerase (RdRp). On the other hand, oral acute toxicity tests demonstrated that HC was non-toxic to laboratory animals following oral administration at 16 g/kg [10].

Jin Yin Hua has protective activity against LPS-induced Lung inflammatory cytokine release. Anti-inflammatory cytokine, IL-10, may prove beneficial in the treatment of endotoxin-associated Lung inflammation [11].

Chai Hu: Chai Hu (Bupleurum Root) is bitter in flavor, slightly cold in nature, and acts on Liver and Gallbladder. It is widely used for the syndromes of wind-heat, Shaoyang syndrome, pain and Liver and Gallbladder disorders. The main components of Chai Hu have Saikoside a, b, c and d, a-spinastral, Volatile oil and fatty acid. It works for the treatment of COVID-19 based on the following rationale:

Saikosaponins exhibit immunomodulatory and anti-inflammatory activities. Saikosaponin A dose-dependently inhibits the production of several inflammatory mediators ROS, TNF-a, COX-2, iNOS, and interleukins (IL-6, IL-8, and IL-10) which are responsible for the cytokine storm of severe COVID-19 patients (12). Saikosaponin D could exhibit an anti-proliferative effect in activated T-lymphocyte, in part via suppression of the nucleotide-binding oligomerization domain 2 (NOD2)/NF-κB, NF-AT, and AP-1 MAPK signaling, which plays a role in the severity and mortality of COVID-19[13].

Saikosaponins exhibited antiviral activities against several types of viruses in experimental studies. Saikosaponin A inhibited influenza A virus and reduced Lung immunopathology. Saikosaponin B demonstrated in-vitro antiviral activity against HCoV-229E by inhibiting the viral attachment to cells in a dose-dependent manner, blocking the viral penetration into cells, and interfering with the early stage of viral replication, such as virus absorption and penetration [14]

A molecular docking study demonstrated that Saikosaponin A has a high affinity to bind to a target receptor of the SARS-CoV-2, ACE II receptor [15].

In conclusion, the papers believe that Saiko Saponins are a candidate treatment for COVID-19 owing to their anti-inflammatory, immunomodulatory, and antiviral activities. We recommend future well-designed randomized controlled trials to evaluate the safety and efficacy of Saikosaponins in patients with COVID-19.

Qing Hao: It has been used for centuries for the treatment of clearing heat and eliminating dampness and cooling blood. It is used for fever and chills, and malaria. Artemisinins are sesquiterpene lactones with a peroxide moiety that are isolated from the herb Artemisia annua. Progressively, research has found that artemisinins displayed multiple pharmacological actions against inflammation, viral infections, and cell and tumour proliferation, making it effective against diseases. Moreover, it has displayed a relatively safe toxicity profile. The use of artemisinins against different respiratory diseases has been investigated in Lung cancer models and inflammatory-driven respiratory disorders. These studies revealed the ability of artemisinins in attenuating proliferation, inflammation, invasion, and metastasis, and in inducing apoptosis. Artemisinins can regulate the expression of pro-inflammatory cytokines, nuclear factor-kappa B (NF-κB), matrix metalloproteinases (MMPs), vascular endothelial growth factor (VEGF), promote cell cycle arrest, drive reactive oxygen species (ROS) production, and induce Bak or Bax-dependent or independent apoptosis. In this review, we aim to provide a comprehensive update of the current knowledge of the effects of artemisinins in relation to respiratory diseases to identify gaps that need to be filled while repurposing artemisinins for the treatment of respiratory diseases. In addition, we postulate whether artemisinins can also be repurposed for the treatment of COVID-19 given its anti-viral and anti-inflammatory properties [16]

Artemisia annua extracts significantly inhibited cytopathy caused by SARS-CoV strain BJ001and showed activity against SARS-CoV-2 in Vero-E6 cell-based cytopathic effect screening [17].

The compounds extracted from *A. annua* have been identified to show antiviral activity against SARS-CoV in Vero cell-based CPE/MTS screening. The results provide strong support for the usage of these herbs to treat SARS-CoV infectious diseases [17].

Acupuncture:

As an important part of TCM, acupuncture and moxibustion therapy have made vital contributions in the history of anti-epidemic action in China. Modern clinical and experimental studies have shown that acupuncture and moxibustion therapy can regulate the human immune function, preventing inflammation and infection. In the current epidemic of COVID-19, acupuncture and moxibustion therapy were actively used for both prevention and treatment [18]. According to Guidelines on Acupuncture and Moxibustion Intervention for COVID-19 (second edition) [19], acupuncture and moxibustion intervention was divided into three phases: medical observation phase (suspected cases), clinical treatment phase (confirmed cases), and convalescence phase. In the medical observation phase, the main points were Fengmen (BL12), Feishu (BL13), Pishu (BL20), Hegu (LI4), Quchi (LI11), Chize (LU5), Yuji (LU10), Qihai (CV6), Zusanli

(ST36), and Sanyinjiao (SP6). The purpose was to stimulate the vital qi and the functions of the Lungs and Spleen, enhancing the viscera's defense. During the clinical treatment phase, the main points chosen were as follows: Hegu (LI4), Taichong (LR3), Tiantu (CV22), Chize (LU5), Kongzui (LU6), Zusanli (ST36), Sanyinjiao (SP6), Dazhu (BLll), Fengmen (BLl2), Feishu (BLl3), Xinshu (BLl5), Geshu (BL17), Zhongfu (LU1), Danzhong (CVl7), Qihai (CV6), Guanyuan (CV4), and Zhongwan (CVl2), in order to stimulate the vital qi of the Lungs and Spleen, protect the viscera, and dispel pathogens. In the convalescence phase, the main points were Neiguan (PC6), Zusanli (ST36), Zhongwan (CVl2), Tianshu (ST25), and Qihai (CV6). The aim in this phase is to remove residual virus, restore vitality, and repair the functions of the Lungs and Spleen. Scholars have provided other ideas for prevention and treatment of COVID-19. Lin Shiyu [20] selected Dazhui (DU14), Fengmen (BLl2), Shaoshang (LU11), Yuji (LU10), Lidui (ST45), and Neiting (ST44) can be used as part of a fire needle treatment plan to prevent COVID-19 and relieve patients' symptoms. Liu Kaiping [21] suggested that moxibustion not only effectively prevents and treats COVID-19, but also improves the quality of life of patients. After the comparative induction and analysis of relevant references [22] pointed out that moxibustion on Dazhui (DU14) and Quchi (LI11) could be selected for fever; moxibustion on Dazhui (DU14), Feishu (BL13), and Dingchuan (EX-B1) could be selected for cough; moxibustion on Zusanli (ST36), Guanyuan (CV4), and Qihai (CV6) could be used for fatigue; and moxibustion on Zhongwan (CV12), Zusanli (ST36), and Tianshu (ST25) could be used for upper digestive system discomfort. Besides, Yang [23] suggested that Ren and Du meridian moxibustion can play an important role in the prevention of new COVID-19 infectionsand in preventing recurrence after recovery.

Acupuncture may play a role in the prevention, treatment and rehabilitation of the COVID-19, and relieve the symptoms caused by COVID-19. Acupuncture has been demonstrated to effectively relieve common symptoms in supportive and palliative care, including, anxiety disorders, nausea, insomnia, leukopenia, fatigue as well as vomiting [24][25].

Acupuncture might also effectively treat abdominal pain and abdominal distension [26]. Coyle et al [26] have proposed that acupuncture is an effective therapeutic approach for chronic obstructive pulmonary disease (COPD) associated breathlessness. Possible related symptoms of COVID-19 treated with acupuncture include anxiety disorder, insomnia, leucopenia, fatigue, nausea and vomiting, abdominal pain and abdominal distension, breathlessness [27]. The recent systematic review and meta-analysis show that acupuncture can relieve breathlessness in subjects with advanced diseases [28]. The review papers found acupuncture could relieve the symptoms of discomfort, subsequently improving the physiological function and quality of life of patients with COVID-19 combined with dyspnea [29]. Although there are only a few clinical reports about acupuncture and moxibustion treatment in COVID-19 patients, it is expected to be a safe and effective adjuvant therapy.

Reference:

1. Al-Bari MA. Chloroquine analogues in drug discovery: new directions of uses, mechanisms of actions and toxic manifestations from malaria to multifarious diseases. *J Antimicrob Chemother.* 2015; 70(6): 1608- 1621.

2. Borba MGS, de Almeida Val F, Sampaio VS, et al. Chloroquine diphosphate in two different dosages as adjunctive therapy of hospitalized patients with severe respiratory syndrome in the context of coronavirus (SARS-CoV-2) infection: preliminary safety results of a randomized, double-blinded, phase IIb clinical trial (CloroCovid-19 study).*medRxiv.* 2020. https://doi.org/10.11 01/2020.04.07.20056424).

3. WHO Rapid Evidence Appraisal for COVID-19 Therapies (REACT) Working Group, Sterne JAC, Murthy S, et al. Association between administration of systemic corticosteroids and mortality among critically ill patients with COVID-19: a meta-analysis. *JAMA.* 2020. Available at: https://www.ncbi.nlm. nih.gov/pubmed/32876694.

4. Wadud N, Ahmed N, Mannu Shergil M, et al. Improved survival outcome in SARs-CoV-2 (COVID-19) acute respiratory distress syndrome patients with tocilizumab administration. *medRxiv.* https://doi.org/10.1101/2020.05.13.20100081

5. *Engineering. published online ahead of print, 2020 Feb 28 (Beijing).* https://doi.org/10.1016/j.eng.2020.02.006.

6. http://www.satcm.gov.cn/xinxifabu/ meitibaodao/2020-04-07/14511.html.

7. Zengli Liu, Xiuhui Li, Chunyan Gou. Effect of Jinhua Qinggan granules on novel coronavirus pneumonia in patients. J Tradit Chin Med. 2020 Jun;40(3):467-472. doi: 10.19852/j.cnki. jtcm.2020.03.016.

8. Long Wen, Zhiguo Zhou, Dixuan Jiang. Effect of Xuebijing injection on inflammatory markers and disease outcome of coronavirus disease 2019. Zhonghua Wei Zhong Bing Ji Jiu Yi Xue. 2020 Apr;32(4):426-429. doi: 10.3760/ cma.j.cn121430-20200406-00386.

9. Yanjun Deng, Bowen Liu, Zhenxiang Liu. Study on active compounds from Huoxiang Zhengqi Oral Liquid for prevention of coronavirus disease 2019 (COVID-19) based on network pharmacology and molecular docking. *Chin. Trad. Herbal Drugs; 5(51): 1113-1122, 20200312.)*

10. Lau KM, Lee KM, Koon CM, et al. Immunomodulatory and anti-SARS activities of Houttuynia cordata. J Ethnopharmacol 2008;118(1):79–85.

11. Kao ST, Liu CJ, Yeh CC. Protective, and immunomodulatory effect of flos Lonicerae japonicae by augmenting IL-10 expression in a murine model of acute Lung inflammation. J Ethnopharmacol 2015; 168:108–15.

12. Yuan B., Yang R., Ma Y., et al. A systematic review of the active saikosaponins and extracts isolated from radix bupleuri and their applications. *Pharm Biol.* 2017; 55:620–635. doi: 10.1080/13880209.2016.1262433.

13. Yang H., Chen X., Jiang C., He K., Hu Y. Antiviral and immunoregulatory role against PCV2 in vivo of Chinese herbal medicinal ingredients. *J Vet Res.* 2017;61:405–410. doi: 10.1515/jvetres-2017-0062.

14. Cheng P.-W., Ng L.-T., Chiang L.-C., et al. Antiviral effects of saikosaponins on human coronavirus 229E in vitro. *Clin Exp Pharmacol Physiol.* 2006;33:612–616. doi: 10.1111/j.1440-1681.2006.04415.x.

15. Yan Y.-M., Shen X., Cao Y.-K., et al. Discovery of anti-2019-nCoV agents from Chinese patent drugs via docking screening. *Preprints.* 2020 doi: 10.20944/preprints202002.0254.v1.

16. Dorothy H J Cheong, Daniel WS Tan, Fred WS Wong, et al. Anti-malarial drug, artemisinin and its derivatives for the treatment of respiratory diseases. Pharmacol Res. 2020 Aug;158:104901. doi: 10.1016/j.phrs.2020.104901. Epub 2020 May 13.

17. Li SY, et al. Identification of natural compounds with antiviral activities against SARS-associated coronavirus. *Antivir Res.* 2005.67: 18–23.

18. ZhenYu Zhao, Yanda Li, Liangyun Zhou, et al.Prevention and treatment of COVID-19 using Traditional Chinese Medicine: A review Phytomedicine. 2021 May; 85: 153308. Published online 2020 Aug 20. doi: 10.1016/j.phymed.2020.153308

19. Lin Z.J., Zhang B. Strategy of pharmaceutical care services for clinical Chinese pharmacists in novel coronavirus pneumonia. *China J. Chin. Materia Medica.* 2020 doi: 10.19540/j.cnki. cjcmm.20200211.501.

20. Lin S.Y., Zhang Y.C., Wei Y.Z., Lin G.H. Exploration of fire-needle therapy on coronavirus disease 2019. *Chin. Acupuncture Moxibustion.* 2020 doi: 10.13703/j.0255-2930.20200223-k0007.

21. Liu K.P., Guan D.D., Li L., Ni H., Chen L. Feasibility analysis of moxibustion whole process intervention in the prevention and treatment of COVID-19. *Acta Chin. Med.* 2020

22. Zhang C.L., Li B., Li J.G., Zou S.S., Dong Z.X., Wang X.T. Syndrome differentiation and treatment of COVID-19 based on wenbing theory in chinese medicine. *Acta Chin. Med.* 2020

23. Yang C., Yuan L., Liu C.Y., Shi J.H., Wang P., Luo M.H. Rational use and pharmaceutical care of Chinese patent medicines based on diagnosis and treatment plan for CoronaVirus Disease 2019. *J. Jinan Univ. (Nat. Sci. Med. Ed.)* 2020

24. Vn Trott P, Oei SL, Ramsenthaler C. Acupuncture for breathlessness in advanced diseases: a systematic review and meta-analysis. *J Pain Symptom Manage* 2020;59:327.e3–38.e3.

25. Amorim D, Amado J, Brito I, et al. Acupuncture and electroacupuncture for anxiety disorders: a systematic review of the clinical research. *Complement Ther Clin Pract* 2018;31:31–7.

26. Coyle ME, Shergis JL, Huang ET, et al. Acupuncture therapies for chronic obstructive pulmonary disease: a systematic review of randomized, controlled trials. *Altern Ther Health Med* 2014;20:10–23.

27. Zhang B, Zhang K, Tang Q, et al. Acupuncture for breathlessness in COVID-19: a protocol for systematic review and meta-analysis. *Medicine (Madr)* 2020;99: e20701.

28. Vn Trott P, Oei SL, Ramsenthaler C. Acupuncture for breathlessness in advanced diseases: a systematic review and meta-analysis. *J Pain Symptom Manage* 2020;59:327.e3–38.e3.

29. Yong Chen, Chengcheng Zhu, Zhangmeng Xu, et al. Acupuncture for coronavirus disease 2019: A protocol for systematic review and meta analysis. Medicine. 2020 Oct 2; 99(40): e22231.

www.ingramcontent.com/pod-product-compliance
Lightning Source LLC
Chambersburg PA
CBHW032054020426
42335CB00011B/332